The Nurses' Guide
to Consumer Health
Web Sites

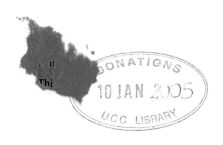

Joyce J. Fitzpatrick, PhD, MBA, RN, FAAN, is Elizabeth Brooks Ford Professor of Nursing, Frances Payne Bolton School of Nursing at Case Western Reserve University in Cleveland, Ohio, where she was Dean from 1982 through 1997. She earned her BSN at Georgetown University, her MS in Psychiatric-Mental Health Nursing at The Ohio State University, her PhD in Nursing at New York University, and an MBA from Case Western Reserve University in 1992. She received the *American Journal of Nursing* Book of the Year Award thirteen times, the Midwest Nursing Research Society Award for Distinguished Contribution to Nursing Research, The Ohio State University Distinguished Alumna Award, the Sigma Theta Tau International Elizabeth McWilliams Miller Founders Award for Excellence in Nursing Research and the New York University Division of Nursing Distinguished Alumna Award. Dr. Fitzpatrick is widely published in nursing and health care literature, having over 250 publications. She is coeditor of the *Annual Review of Nursing Research* series, now in its nineteenth volume, and editor of the journals *Applied Nursing Research* and *Nursing and Health Care Perspectives*. From 1997 to 1999, Dr. Fitzpatrick was the President of the American Academy of Nursing.

Carol A. Romano, PhD, RN, C, CNAA, FAAN, is Deputy Chief, Department of Clinical Research Informatics, Clinical Center, at the National Institutes of Health. She has an undergraduate degree in Nursing, a graduate degree in Administration/Nursing, and a PhD with a focus on Operations Analysis/Informatics from the University of Maryland. Dr. Romano is also a Commissioned Officer with the senior rank of Captain in the Nurse Corps of the U.S. Public Health Service. Her accomplishments at NIH have been recognized with the NIH Director's Award, the PHS Meritorious Medal, Outstanding Service Medal, Commendation Medal, Achievement Medal, and several citations. She has authored over 50 professional published papers and holds a university faculty appointment at University of Maryland. She has also served as chair of the Commission on Certification of the American Nurses Credentialing Center, member of the USPDI Advisory Board on Therapeutic Information Management, and co-chair of the Maryland State Board of Nursing Task Force on Standards of Practice.

Ruth Chasek has been Nursing Editor at Springer Publishing Company for over 15 years, where she has worked on many award-winning books.

The Nurses' Guide to Consumer Health Web Sites

Joyce J. Fitzpatrick, PhD, RN, FAAN
Carol Romano, PhD, RN, FAAN
Ruth Chasek, Editors

 Springer Publishing Company

Copyright © 2001 by Springer Publishing Company, Inc.

Springer Publishing Company, Inc.
536 Broadway
New York, NY 10012-3955

Acquisitions Editor: Ruth Chasek
Production Editor: J. Hurkin-Torres
Cover design by Susan Hauley

03 04 05 / 5 4

Library of Congress Cataloging-in-Publication Data

The nurses' guide to consumer health web sites / [edited by] Joyce J. Fitzpatrick, Carol Romano, Ruth Chasek.
   p. ; cm.
   Includes bibliographical references and index.
   ISBN 0-8261-1455-5
   1. Nursing—Computer network resources.   2. Internet.   3. Web sites.   4. Medical care—Computer network resources.   I. Fitzpatrick, Joyce J., 1944–.   II. Romano, Carol Ann.   III. Chasek, Ruth.
   [DNLM: 1. Internet—Nurses' Instruction.   2. Patient Education—methods—Nurses' Instruction.   3. Health Promotion—methods—Nurses' Instruction. WY 26.5 N97315 2001]
   RT50.5 .N85 2001
   025.06'61073—dc21   2001040001
                                                                           CIP

Printed in Canada

To Liddy, who encouraged this endeavor, and to my daughters
Maria and Regina

JJF

To my mother, Mary, for her continued love and
encouragement

CAR

To Dad, who always prefers self-help, and to my whole family

RMC

Contents

Part IV.   Negotiating the Health Care System

Contributors

Devon Berry, MSN, RN, CFNP
Assistant Professor
Department of Nursing
Cedarville University
Cedarville, OH

Jacquelyn C. Campbell, PhD, RN, FAAN
Anna D. Wolf Endowed Professor
Associate Dean for PhD Program and Research
School of Nursing
The Johns Hopkins University
Baltimore, MD

Kathryn Chouaf, MSN, RN
PhD Candidate
School of Nursing
The Johns Hopkins University
Baltimore, MD

Joseph P. Colagreco, MS, RN, ANP-CS
Clinical Assistant Professor
Division of Nursing
New York University
New York, NY
Clinical Manager
Infectious Disease Clinic
Mount Sinai Medical Center
New York, NY

Sarah P. Farrell, PhD, RN, CS
UVA Shaughnessy Fellow
School of Nursing
University of Virginia
Charlottesville, VA

Sandra A. Faux, PhD, RN
Associate Professor
Maternal Child Nursing Department
College of Nursing
Rush University
Chicago, IL

Betty J. Furr, MSN, RN, CRRN
Clinical Nurse Manager, Brain Injury Unit
Neuroscience and Restorative Care Center
Mount Sinai Medical Center
New York, NY

Jill M. Goldstein, MA, MS, RN
Clinical Nurse Manager
Mount Sinai Medical Center
New York, NY

Patricia G. Hinegardner, MLS, AHIP
Coordinator of Specialized Information Services
Health Sciences and Human Services Library
University of Maryland
Baltimore, MD

Angela L. Hudson, PhD, RN
Postdoctoral Fellow
Department of Community Health Systems
School of Nursing
University of California San Francisco
San Francisco, CA

Trudy Johnson, MA, RN, CNAA
Director of Performance Improvement
  Services
New York–Presbyterian Hospital
New York, NY

Sandra Jones, MA, RN
Professor
John Tyler Community College
Richmond, VA

Françoise Juste, BSN, RNC
Clinical Nurse, Surgical Intensive Care
  Unit
Mount Sinai Medical Center
New York, NY

**Carl A. Kirton, MA, RN, ANP-CS,
  ACRN**
Clinical Assistant Professor of Nursing
Division of Nursing
New York University
New York, NY
Clinical Manager
Infectious Disease Clinic
Mount Sinai Medical Center
New York, NY

**Felissa R. Lashley, PhD, RN, ACRN,
  FAAN**
Dean and Professor
School of Nursing
Southern Illinois
  University—Edwardsville
Edwardsville, IL

Kathryn A. Lee, PhD, RN, FAAN
Professor
Department of Family Health Care
  Nursing
School of Nursing
University of California—San
  Francisco
San Francisco, CA

Dorothy Lemmey, PhD, RN
Assistant Professor
School of Nursing
University of Maryland
Baltimore, MD

Kim Malusis, MS, RN, FNP
Nurse Practitioner
Mount Sinai Medical Center
New York, NY

**Marianne LaPorte Matzo, PhD, RN,
  CS, GNP**
Professor of Nursing
New Hampshire Community Technical
  College
Manchester, NH

**Graham J. McDougall, Jr., PhD, RN,
  CS**
Associate Professor
School of Nursing
The University of Texas at Austin
Austin, Texas

Kathleen M. McPhaul, MPH, RN
Doctoral Student
Department of Community and
  Behavioral Health
School of Nursing
University of Maryland
Baltimore, MD

Rita G. Mertig, MS, RNC, CNS
Professor of Nursing
John Tyler Community College
Chester, VA

Ethel L. Mitty, EdD, RN
Research Associate and Adjunct
  Assistant Professor
Division of Nursing
New York University
New York, NY

Kristen S. Montgomery, PhD, RNC, IBCLC
Postdoctoral Fellow
School of Nursing
University of Michigan
Ann Arbor, MI

Karen H. Morin, DSN, RN
Professor of Nursing and
Professor in Charge of Graduate
Programs
School of Nursing
The Pennsylvania State University
University Park, PA

Georgia L. Narsavage, PhD, RN, CS
Associate Professor and Director of
the MSN Program
Frances Payne Bolton School of
Nursing
Case Western Reserve University
Cleveland, OH

Wendy M. Nehring, PhD, RN
Associate Professor and Director of
Undergraduate Programs
School of Nursing
Southern Illinois
University—Edwardsville
Edwardsville, IL

Linda J. O'Connor, MSN, RNC, CS
Gerontological Clinical Nurse
Specialist
Project Coordinator
Nursing Care Quality Initiative
North Shore–Long Island Jewish
Health System and
Mount Sinai NYU Health
Manhasset, NY

Ann L. O'Sullivan, PhD, RN, FAAN, CPNP
Associate Professor of Pediatric
Primary Care Nursing
Director, Pediatric Nurse Practitioner
Program
School of Nursing
University of Pennsylvania
Philadelphia, PA

Linda Peters, MS, RN, CPNP
Nurse Practitioner
Mount Sinai Medical Center
New York, NY

Cynthia R. Phyillaier, MSLS
Information Specialist and Liaison to
School of Nursing
Health Sciences and Human Services
Library
University of Maryland
Baltimore, MD

Nancy E. Reame, PhD, RN, FAAN
Rhetaugh Graves Dumas Endowed
Professor of Nursing
Research Scientist, Reproductive
Sciences Program
School of Nursing
University of Michigan
Ann Arbor, MI

Audrey J. Schmerzler, MSN, RN, CRRN
Nurse Clinician
Mount Sinai School of Medicine
New York, NY

Cynthia A. Schmidt, PhD, RN
Assistant Professor
School of Nursing
Southern Illinois
University—Edwardsville
Edwardsville, IL

Laree J. Schoolmeesters, MSN, RN
Doctoral Candidate
Frances Payne Bolton School of
Nursing
Case Western Reserve University
Cleveland, OH

Meg Smirnoff, MPH, RN, FNP
Clinical Coordinator
Pediatric Asthma Program
Mount Sinai Medical Center
New York, NY

Mariah Snyder, PhD, RN, FAAN
Professor
School of Nursing
University of Minnesota
Minneapolis, MN

Hussein A. Tahan, MS, RN, CNA
Director of Nursing, Cardiac
  Specialties
New York–Presbyterian Hospital
Columbia Presbyterian Medical Center
New York, NY

Kristine M. C. Talley, BSN, RN
Community Program Specialist
Fall Evaluation and Prevention
  Program
School of Nursing
University of Minnesota
Minneapolis, MN

Diana L. Taylor, PhD, RN, FAAN
Associate Professor
Department of Family Health Care
  Nursing
School of Nursing
University of California—San
  Francisco
San Francisco, CA

Dorothy C. Visco, BSN, RN, CWCN
Wound Care Specialist
Mount Sinai Hospital Home Health
  Agency
New York, NY

Gina M. Wade, MS, RN
Assistant Clinical Professor
School of Nursing
University of California—San
  Francisco
San Francisco, CA

Meredith Wallace, PhD, RN, CS-ANP
Assistant Professor
Department of Nursing
Southern Connecticut State University
New Haven, CT

Jane Weiser, EdD, RN, IBCLC
Nurse Clinician, Lactation Consultant,
  and Childbirth Educator
Mount Sinai Hospital
New York, NY

**Susan J. Wren, BSN, RN, CWCN,
COCN**
Wound/Ostomy Care Nurse
New York–Presbyterian Hospital
  Home Health Agency
New York, NY

**Jean F. Wyman, PhD, RN, CS,
FAAN**
Professor and Cora Meidl Siehl Chair
  in Nursing Research
School of Nursing
University of Minnesota
Minneapolis, MN

Introduction

This book gives both the professional and the patient a tool for finding reliable health information on the Internet. The sites in this book have been selected and reviewed by expert nurses in 40 specialties, most of them nursing educators with doctoral degrees. The result is a treasure of information sources, which can be used for health promotion, preventive care, or enhancing one's understanding of a medical condition.

The Web sites chosen are chiefly those of major institutions, both government and private, that have created these sites as an extension of the missions of their institutions, which have long preceded the Internet. However, because the Internet is everchanging, consumers should be aware of ways to evaluate new and unfamiliar information on the Web that they may encounter.

Several organizations and groups have identified criteria for evaluating Web sites. One such organization is the Health on the Net (HON) Foundation (*http://www.hon.ch*). Sites that meet its Code of Conduct are often designated by the "HON Code" symbol. Our comparison of several different sources that suggest evaluation criteria yielded five common criteria for evaluation. These criteria are the following:

- *Authority/Source:* The author or organization should be identified. If it is a person, what are his or her credentials or experience with the subject? If it is an organization, is it reputable? Is there a way to contact the authors or sponsors of the site?
- *Purpose/Objectivity:* Is the purpose of the site clearly stated? Who is the intended audience? If there is sponsorship, is it fully disclosed?
- *Content:* Is the information accurate, useful, and relevant to the needs of the audience? Is the scope appropriate? Are selection criteria included? Are there relevant and authoritative links? Is factual information verifiable? Are spelling and grammar accurate?
- *Currency:* Is the production date clearly indicated? Are revision dates included? Are links up to date?

- *Design:* Is the site well organized and easy to navigate? Are graphics meaningfully used, or do they clutter the screen? Is the site stable?

ABOUT THE BOOK

The book is divided into four key parts. Part I includes a review of the general health and medical Web sites. These sites cover a range of topics and offer a great deal of information on many health conditions. They also provide links to other sites and often lead the consumer to specialty sites and other resources, such as additional sources of information, support groups, and statistical resources. Part II includes a review of the drug information and medication sites.

Part III includes a review of special topics. In preparing the list of topics to be included in this section, we asked ourselves these questions: What health conditions are so common in their occurrence that individuals would look for information on the Internet? What are the common health-related questions that may occur independent of illness? Thus, in this section we have included three types of sites: disease topics, such as diabetes mellitus; conditions, such as fatigue; and health promotion/disease prevention information, such as travel considerations, exercise and physical fitness, and diet, nutrition, and weight loss.

Part IV gives sites that are important resources for those negotiating the health care system. Included here are reviews of sites such as home care services and long-term care services.

HOW THE SITES WERE CHOSEN

The authors were chosen based on their expertise in a given field of nursing and health care. Consistent criteria were used by each author in evaluating the sites for inclusion. Specifically, the authors were asked to select the top 1–6 sites in their area of expertise and to review these sites for relevance to consumer use. They were told to select sites that would be most useful to consumers looking for health information. The authors then provided the following information, based on the evaluation criteria discussed above:

1. A brief overall description of the site
2. A statement of the purpose of the site

3. Sponsors of the site
4. Intended audience of the site
5. Currency and accuracy of the information on the site
6. Most important features of the site
7. Any weak points of the site
8. Whether or not the site information is available in any language in addition to English
9. Overall rating level of the information available through the site
10. Comments on the site's appearance and ease of use

TO OUR READERS

We use the term *consumers* throughout the book to describe individuals seeking health information, not in the sense of savvy shoppers, but in the sense of users—in this case, users of knowledge.

We also assume a general level of proficiency in Internet use by the reader. However, the Internet will always have novice users. To help get over the "bump" of your first encounters with the Web, we recommend that you consult a tutorial site such as "Web Teacher" (*http://www.webteacher.org*).

We believe that this book will be very useful to health professionals everywhere. More importantly, we are aware of the even greater need to reach consumers with accurate, timely, and useful health care information provided at their fingertips through the Internet. This book serves as an important step toward achieving that goal.

JOYCE J. FITZPATRICK
CAROL A. ROMANO
RUTH CHASEK

Part **I**

The Megasites

Chapter 1

General Health and Medical Web Sites*

Carol A. Romano, PhD, RN, C, CNAA, FAAN,
Cynthia R. Phyillaier, MSLS, and
Patricia G. Hinegardner, MLS, AHIP

Although the Internet provides a rich source of health information to nurses, health care professionals, and the general public, it also poses many challenges. Which sites can be relied on for reliable and quality information? Which sites can health professionals safely recommend to their patients? Recent studies (Biermann, Golla-day, Greenfield, & Baker, 1999; Schloman, 1999) have noted erroneous information found on some consumer health Web sites. Criteria are needed to evaluate Internet sites to protect against fraudulent claims, inaccurate information, and potential harm.

This chapter describes eight "megasites" providing consumer health information in general health and medical care. The methodology used to select these sites included (1) selection of evaluation criteria and (2) identification of sites referenced in the literature that met these criteria. The selection of review criteria was made from a literature search of the authoritative databases of MEDLINE and CINAHL. A comparison of sources yielded five common criteria:

- authority and credibility of source
- purpose and objectivity
- content accuracy and relevancy

---

*This chapter is in the public domain. It was prepared by employees of the state and federal government and cannot be copyrighted.

- currency
- design

A second literature search identified articles that evaluated specific sites. The "megasites" presented in this chapter were reviewed by more than one reference and met the criteria identified above. It is noted, however, that Web sites are dynamic and change over time. The eight Web sites below are listed in alphabetical order.

Centers for Disease Control and Prevention

http://www.cdc.gov

The Centers for Disease Control and Prevention (CDC), an agency of the U.S. Department of Health and Human Services, is comprised of 11 centers, institutes, and offices dedicated to promoting "health and quality of life by preventing and controlling disease, injury, and disability." The Web site provides access to health information and statistics produced by the various entities within the organization. The site offers information for both the health professional and the consumer.

Of special interest to consumers are the resources on diseases, conditions, and other special topics that are gleaned from the general CDC Web site. These resources are arranged alphabetically under "Health Topics A–Z." New topics are continuously being added, and update information or "last reviewed" dates appear on many of the resources. The Web site also includes a section on "Hoaxes and Rumors," which describes bogus information that may be found on the Internet or from other sources of communication. The "Travelers' Health" section contains worldwide health recommendations for travelers by geographic location and disease outbreaks. Vaccine recommendations are provided for individual countries.

Navigating the site is easy. The content list provides access to the major sections of the Web site, and keyword searching is also available. Because the 11 branches of the CDC design their own sites, there is variability in the format and content of the subject matter covered. A Spanish-language section targets information to specific interest groups, such as students, adolescents, and women, and provides information by health topic. There is also a "Contact Us" link, which provides an e-mail address and toll-free number for public inquiries and feedback.

Healthfinder

http://www.healthfinder.gov

Developed by the Office of Disease Prevention and Health Promotion, U.S. Department of Health and Human Services, with other listed agencies, Healthfinder is a gateway to consumer health information. The goal of the site is "to improve consumer access to selected health information from government agencies, their many partner organizations, and other reliable sources that serve the public interest." It provides links to online journals, medical dictionaries, and information on minority health and prevention and self-care. The target audience is the general public, but health professionals will also find the site useful.

A steering committee of representatives of federal agencies, nonfederal consumer health information specialists, and librarians coordinates the site. Information for over 1,400 organizations is linked using selected guidelines that are identified at the site. The currency of information varies depending on the host organization.

There are six major sections: "Hot Topics" highlights monthly top search topics and favorites; "News" provides health news and acts as a gateway to government, professional, and Web news media; "Smart Choices" provides links to resources in the areas of prevention and self-care, choosing quality care, online health information, and fraud and complaints; "More Tools" provides access to libraries, medical dictionaries, support groups, and so on; "Just for You" includes information by age group, men and women, and special populations (a Spanish-language section is available); and "About Us" provides information about Healthfinder, including selection criteria.

Healthfinder is easy to navigate. Searching may be done either by typing in search terms using the keyword search option or by selecting a link from within one of the major sections. A typical entry under a disease includes a list of specific Web resources and a list of organizations that gives further information on the condition. A useful feature in these listings is the "Details" option that provides information about the site being accessed.

HealthWeb

http://healthweb.org

HealthWeb was established by librarians and information professionals from major academic medical institutions in the Midwest. It is a collaborative project of the health sciences libraries of the Greater Midwest Region (GMR) of the National Network of Libraries of Medicine (NN/ LM) and those of the Committee for Institutional Cooperation. The HealthWeb project was conceived in 1994 with the goal of developing "an interface which will provide organized access to evaluated non-commercial, health-related, Internet-accessible resources" (Redman et al., 1997). HealthWeb is a tool to facilitate access to quality health-related resources on the Internet. Information specialists collect, evaluate, and organize health information and education resources for health care professionals and consumers. Each library participating in the project is responsible for maintaining and updating its selected area. This includes a regular review of links to make sure they are current and to update any locally mounted information on a regular basis.

An alphabetical list of diseases and health-related topics is displayed on the main page of the site. Resources within a topic are organized into categories. For example, under Oncology the categories include Academic Institutes and Research Groups, Clinical Resources, Clinical Trials, Conferences, Consumer Health Resources, and Statistics. Categories will vary depending on the topic. After choosing a category, there is an option to choose a "Long Display" that includes very brief descriptions of the sites listed. A keyword search feature allows for searching within the specific topic area or the entire HealthWeb site.

The site also provides "User Guides" developed to help health care professionals and consumers use Internet resources more effectively. The guides include "Evaluating Internet Resources," "Searching the Internet," and "Document Delivery." A "FeedBack" link gives users the opportunity to provide general feedback about the site, report a dead link, or suggest a site to add to HealthWeb.

MayoClinic.com

http://www.mayoclinic.com

MayoClinic.com (formerly the Mayo Clinic Health Oasis) is an excellent source of consumer health information. The site is compiled by a staff of over 2,000 people who are physicians, scientists, nurses, writers, and educators at the Mayo Clinic, a nonprofit institution. The site's mission is to help people find answers to manage illness and to stay healthy. Although its purpose is educational, *MayoClinic.com* does include some advertising by commercial sponsors. Ads are kept to a minimum and must meet strict guidelines. The editorial policy states that Mayo does not endorse any company or product (Rogers, 1998). The site's original format has been expanded considerably with its new name. In addition to the major centers of health information that existed previously (e.g., Allergy & Asthma, Arthritis, and Cancer), interactive applications and tools to assist consumers in managing their health have made the site more comprehensive. Of the three major sections of the site, "Find Information," "Take Charge of Your Health," and "Connect with Others," the second two are new. "Take Charge of Your Health" includes a Personal Health Scorecard, Healthy Lifestyle Planners, Disease Self-Managers, and Health Decision Guides. They present a series of multiple-choice questions, then tailor results based on the responses entered. "Connect with Others" was not available at press time but will provide the following options when operational: Member-to-Member Forums, Health e-Conferences, and Chat with a Mayo Specialist. A free, weekly e-mail newsletter, "Housecall," which includes new health and fitness information, is available to anyone who wishes to subscribe.

Another significant new feature of the site is "My Mayo." This allows an individual to choose preferences in a "My Mayo Profile," which is then used to select and display articles on subjects of interest to that individual. The feature also allows saving of specific articles and pages to a "My Mayo Bookshelf" area for easy retrieval.

A "Drug Name" search box continues to be available on the homepage for searching by generic or brand-name drugs in the *USP Drug Guide* for consumers. A "Contact Us" feature allows consumers to e-mail questions to physicians or dietitians.

The site is well designed and user-friendly but more cluttered than previously. It is easy to navigate, and those few advertisements that appear do not interfere with the content of the site. As might be expected with a site that permits individual health profiling and interactivity, *MayoClinic.com* requires registration for security reasons. There is no fee to register, and the user must agree to an extensive online agreement and privacy policy. Information at *MayoClinic.com* is timely and accurate. The site is updated every weekday, and all material is dated.

Medem

http://www.medem.com

Medem is a project of the leading medical societies in the United States. The founding societies include the American Medical Association (AMA), the American Academy of Ophthalmology, the American Academy of Pediatrics, the American College of Allergy, Asthma, and Immunology, the American College of Obstetricians and Gynecologists, the American Psychiatric Association, and the American Society of Plastic Surgeons. The site was developed to provide "a trusted online source for credible, comprehensive, and clinical health care information, and secure, confidential communications."

Medem has launched various services, including "Your Practice Online," which allows physicians to create a practice Web site; "Medex Secure Messaging," which permits patients and physicians to interact in a secure communications environment; and the "Medical Library," which contains health care information for both consumers and health care professionals. Information in Medem is provided and approved by the participating medical societies, making it an excellent source of information for consumers.

The "Medical Library" is divided into four major categories: Life Stages; Diseases and Conditions; Therapies and Health Strategies; and Health and Society. These categories are further subdivided. For example, Therapies and Health Strategies includes Preventive Medicine, Fitness and Nutrition, Complementary and Alternative Medicine, Plastic Surgery, Medical Tests and Medications, Pain Management, and Physical Medicine and Rehabilitation. A list of document titles displays under a specific topic. Next to each title is an icon that indicates whether the information provided is introductory, general, advanced, or at the professional/research level. Information sources range from peer-reviewed journal articles to medical news. Dates are listed on the resources.

The site is well organized and easy to use. Users can browse through the site using the category links or search the site using the text box provided. An advanced search feature that allows a search to be refined by a specific category and then sorted by relevance or source is available on the "Medical Library" page. A "Search Tips" link offers suggestions for searching.

The site also has a link to the "AMA Physician Finder." This service allows users to locate a physician in a geographic area by specialty or name. A "Contact Us" link provides a toll-free phone number and an e-mail address for comments.

MEDLINEplus

http://www.medlineplus.gov

MEDLINEplus is a consumer-oriented Web site established in 1998 by the National Library of Medicine (NLM), the world's largest biomedical library. The NLM staff of information experts select and revise the content from governmental and nongovernmental publications, brochures, databases, and Web sites. The NLM is part of the National Institutes of Health (NIH), an agency of the Department of Health and Human Services. The site's purpose is to provide accurate and current medical information to anyone with a medical question. Although the site targets consumers, health care professionals will find useful information here.

Information can be obtained by selecting from an alphabetical list, labeled "Health Topics," which consists of over three hundred specific diseases, conditions, and wellness issues. Individual topics are covered with reliable resources that are unrivaled in subject comprehensiveness (O'Leary, 2000). Each "Health Topic" page contains links to authoritative information on that subject, as well as an optional link to a preformulated MEDLINE database search with results on that subject. Because a study by the NLM in 1998 of MEDLINE utilization statistics determined that 30% of the database searches were performed by members of the general public, access to MEDLINE was included at this site (Miller, Lacroix, & Backus, 2000). MEDLINE consists of citations with abstracts to eleven million research articles published in 4,300 biomedical journals and is considered the "gold standard" of medical databases. By having the search results preformulated, the consumer does not have to know special searching techniques to retrieve useful information from the database. An alternate method for locating information on a particular subject is a search box in which a word or phrase is entered.

MEDLINEplus is much more than results from the MEDLINE database because it provides a number of additional resources. There are many useful directories that include locations and credentials of hospitals, doctors, and other health care providers. A list to several online medical dictionaries provides access to definitions of unfamiliar medical terms. Drug information for consumers is available from the United States Pharmacopeia in easily understood terms and can be searched either by generic or brand name. A number of resources listed at the site include links to full text publications available from the NIH and other governmental and nongovernmental organizations.

MEDLINEplus is easy to navigate. There are no advertisements or cluttered graphics obscuring the information. The homepage and major sections of the site can be quickly accessed without having to go through multiple "back" buttons. Each Health Topic page displays the release date for that topic, and all sections of the site are continuously updated. New health topics are frequently added, most recently one on West Nile virus. An automatic link checker is in place, and broken links are corrected on a daily basis to ensure currency of information. A Spanish-language format is also available.

New York Online Access to Health

http://www.noah-health.org

The New York Online Access to Health (NOAH) is one of the oldest established consumer health sites on the Web. Launched in 1995, it is comprised of a collection of state, local, and federal resources selected by volunteer librarian/editors with the assistance of a scientific advisory board consisting of interdisciplinary health professionals (Voge, 1998). The mission of NOAH, "to provide high quality full-text information for consumers that is accurate, timely, relevant and unbiased," is clearly accomplished with the current site. The original four site sponsors, the City University of New York, the New York Academy of Medicine, the New York Public Library, and the Metropolitan New York Library Council, have been joined in recent years by additional sponsors, the majority of whom are libraries.

NOAH is unique in that it is completely bilingual. This reflects another of NOAH's stated goals: to provide an "authoritative bilingual health information site, dedicated to an underserved population of health consumers, many of whom are also Spanish speaking." Consumers can access all menus and resources beginning from the site's homepage.

Content includes a number of broad "Health Topics," which are arranged alphabetically and then broken into numerous subcategories to include definitions, care and treatment, and lists of information resources. Sources are linked to content. For example, the content on the basics of diabetes is linked to full text items by the American Diabetes Association, the Joslin Diabetes Center, and the Merck Manual. The quality and depth of the sites chosen provide consumers with much needed information in terms that they can comprehend. A disclaimer is also provided that identifies NOAH as an information guide that should not be interpreted as professional or medical advice.

NOAH is designed with the easy navigability required by the novice user. A directory format allows selection of broad health categories that lead to more specific subcategories. For those who prefer to search by text word(s), an alternate method of searching is a word search, in which a word or phrase is typed into a text box. The word search at NOAH uses the Excite search engine; however, it only searches documents located at the NOAH site. Information is presented in a clear and logical manner throughout, and there are no advertisements.

U.S. Consumer Gateway: Health

http://www.consumer.gov/health.htm

The U.S. Consumer Gateway is a true megasite for consumer information from the federal government. The site's purpose is to provide a one-stop link to a range of federal resources on the Web easily available to consumers. It is designed so that information can be located by category; "Health" is one of 10 broad categories at this gateway site.

The site consists of links to dozens of participating federal agencies, including the Agency for Healthcare Research and Quality, the Centers for Disease Control, the Food and Drug Administration, the National Institutes of Health, the National Library of Medicine, and the Occupational Safety and Health Administration. Information links are arranged under eight broad health categories (e.g., "Choosing Quality Health Care," "Drugs," and "Exercise and Fitness"), and each link lists the source federal agency. In addition to the eight major health categories, there is a list of recent information links in the "In the Spotlight" section on the front page. There are also links to the "Healthfinder" and "Healthy People 2010" gateways, and many of the disease links lead to subject areas in the MEDLINEplus site. Content is selected with the consumer in mind. Under the category "Choosing Quality Health Care," there is a link to "Consumer Versions of Clinical Practice Guidelines."

The site is designed for ease of navigation without frames and time-consuming graphics. Each document displays its originating agency, and documents are arranged alphabetically within each broad health category. Revision dates are posted for items on the site, and the "Health" section appears to be updated at least once a week. The majority of data from the site is in English, with occasional links to resources in other languages (e.g., Spanish). An extensive Privacy Policy reassures consumers that their information-seeking rights are protected at the site.

ADDITIONAL MEGASITE

The Merck Manual—Home Edition

http://www.merck.homeedition.com

See review in Chapter 39, "Understanding Medical Jargon."

REFERENCES

Biermann, J., Golladay, G., Greenfield, M. L., & Baker, L. (1999). Evaluation of cancer information on the Internet. *Cancer, 86,* 381–390.

Miller, N., Lacroix, E. M., & Backus, J. E. (2000). MEDLINEplus: Building and maintaining the National Library of Medicine's consumer health Web service. *Bulletin of the Medical Library Association, 88,* 11–17.

O'Leary, M. (2000). MEDLINEplus: MEDLINE for the masses. *Information Today, 17,* 20–21.

Redman, P. M., Kelly, J. A., Albright, E. D., Anderson, P. F., Mulder, C., & Schnell, E. H. (1997). Common ground: The HealthWeb project as a model for Internet collaboration. *Bulletin of the Medical Library Association, 85,* 325–330.

Rogers, A. (1998). Good medicine on the Web. *Newsweek, 132,* 60.

Schloman, B. F. (1999). Whom do you trust? Evaluating Internet health resources. *Online Journal of Issues in Nursing.* Accessed October 13, 1999. Available at http://www.nursingworld.org.ojin/infocol/info_1.htm.

Setton, D. (2000). Here's to your health. *Forbes, 165,* 118.

Voge, S. (1998). NOAH—New York online access to health: Library collaboration for bilingual consumer health information on the Internet. *Bulletin of the Medical Library Association, 86,* 326–334.

Part **II**

Medications

Chapter 2

Drug Information and Medications

Kristen S. Montgomery, PhD, RNC, IBCLC

At some point in one's life, almost everyone receives a prescription medication for an illness, infection, or other condition. Some individuals are prescribed medication that will be needed for a lifetime, others for only a brief period of time. Whatever the type, dose, or frequency of the medication, the person taking it needs to understand why they have been prescribed the medication, what the medication is intended to do, and if there are any side effects associated with using the medication. Consumers also need to be aware of any precautions that need to be followed while taking the medication and precisely how to take the medication for maximum benefit. Web sites that provide quality information for consumers are provided within this section.

FDA Information for Consumers

http://www.fda.gov/opacom/morecons.html

FDA Consumer Drug Information Page

http://www.fda.gov/cder/consumerinfo

The FDA Information for Consumers Page is an information resource for consumers on all products regulated by the U.S. Food and Drug Administration: foods, dietary supplements, prescription and non-prescription medications, medical devices, veterinary medical products, and cosmetics. Information is accurate and current. The most important features of the site are the broad categories that become more specific when the user clicks on the section. The prescription drug section is *The FDA Consumer Drug Information Page* (one can directly access this page with the address listed above). This profiles drugs approved by the U.S. Food and Drug Administration (FDA) since 1998 in an easy-to-understand format, with information on active ingredients, dosage, usage, and precautions. It is an excellent resource for consumers seeking brief and accessible knowledge on new drugs. However, one should note that many common drugs produced before 1998 will not be on this page. The date content was last revised is noted at the bottom of each drug profile. The non-prescription drug section includes general guidelines on drug usage, reading labels, drug interactions, pregnancy and breastfeeding information, considerations with children, and protection against tampering, but it does not describe specific over-the-counter drugs. Text is available in English and is easy to use. Information is presented at an average level.

Health-Center.com Pharmacy

http://www1.health-center.com/pharmacy

Health-Center.com Pharmacy is the pharmacy section of a larger Web site. It is a comprehensive site for medication information that is geared toward consumers. The site is sponsored by Health-Center.com, which was created by Clinical Tools, Inc., a physician-owned, multi-media company located in Chapel Hill, North Carolina, and Pittsburgh, Pennsylvania. The site is intended for consumers and provides current and accurate information. Medications are sorted by category (e.g., anti-anxiety, Alzheimer's) and within each category common drugs for the category are listed. The user can click on the drug of their choice and find out more detailed information, including common uses of the drug, when the drug will start to work, and side effects. Side effects are identified as most common, infrequent, and rare. Drug interaction concerns are also noted. In addition, there are mechanisms to email an entire page, provide feedback, and format the page for printing. Discussion groups are also coordinated via the Web site. No weak points were noted. The site is available in English at a simple level. It is easy to use.

MayoClinic.com

http://www.mayoclinic.com

MEDLINEplus

http://www.nlm.nih.gov/medlineplus

WebMD Health

http://mywebmd.com

All of these major health Web sites, and many others, feature the same drug information database—"USPDI Advice for the Patient," which is licensed from Micromedex, a software publishing company. Micromedex is owned by publishing giant Thomson. The database is produced under the supervision of The United States Pharmacopeial Convention (USP), a nonprofit, nongovernment organization that sets standards for drug products in the United States. The information in the Micromedex database has been formatted in a user-friendly, consumer-oriented style, with a 12th grade reading level. Material is presented in four to eight pages, including brand name, purpose, description, proper use, precautions, and side effects. The date description was developed is noted. Information is in English. This is an authoritative source of information in a readable style, which must be why so many Web sites have adopted it.

Medication Information Index

http://www.cheshire-med.com/services/pharm/medindex.html

Medication Information Index is a resource page for consumers who need information regarding commonly prescribed medications. The site is sponsored by The Cheshire Medical Center, which is located in Keene, New Hampshire. Information within the site is current and accurate. The site is arranged alphabetically to enhance the user's ability to locate a specific medication. A local phone number is also provided for consumers that have additional questions. The site is linked to a search engine. Generic and trade names are provided. The site is only available in English and information is presented at a simple level.

National Institute on Aging Age Page, Medicines: Use Them Safely

http://www.aoa.dhhs.gov/aoa/pages/agepages/medicine.html

This site is a one-page description of how to safely use medications in the elderly. People over the age of 65 take 25% of all prescription drugs, and these drugs may affect them differently than younger people. The site is sponsored by the Institute of Aging for the purpose of providing information to elderly consumers and their family members. It is not drug-specific, but has useful tips and suggestions like crushing pills if one has difficulty swallowing. It also includes a prepared list of questions one can ask a doctor. Information is accurate and current. Text is provided in English at a simple to average level.

Not-2-Late.Com: The Emergency Contraception Website

http://ec.princeton.edu

Not-2-Late.Com is a comprehensive resource on emergency contraception that is geared toward consumers. The site is sponsored by The Office of Population Research at Princeton University. The information provided on the site is accurate and current. The site is easy to use and includes information on what emergency contraception is, different types of emergency contraception available, health care providers who dispense emergency contraception, frequently asked questions, and information on the peer review panel. There is also reference information and global statistics on emergency contraception use. The site is available in English, Spanish, and French. Information is presented at an average level and the site is easy to use.

RxList

http://www.rxlist.com

RxList is an information resource intended primarily for health professionals. It is useful to consumers because of the detailed listing of drug ingredients, including inactive ingredients. This is invaluable to those who are allergic to common "fillers" like lactose. Included with the description of each drug is information on usage, warnings, precautions, adverse reactions, drug interactions, and overdose. Interesting sections include a list of the top 200 most frequently prescribed drugs and drug specific discussions. RxList also features sections on alternative medicine, an online store, patient education materials, and related links.

The site was founded and is maintained by Neil Sandow, PharmD. It is a Health Central Network site. Health Central.com is a commercial, publicly traded company, founded in 1998, that provides online health care content and ecommerce.

Overall this is a good site. The page is well organized, but appears a bit cluttered. The site is very comprehensive. A negative feature is the advertisements that are not pharmacy or health care related.

Part **III**

Special Topics

Chapter 3

Adolescents

Ann L. O'Sullivan, PhD, RN, FAAN, CPNP

The following Web sites have been selected based on their extensive links to current resources about the health of adolescents. In addition, each of the Web sites provides a listing and brief description of publications and ordering information.

Advocates for Youth

http://www.advocatesforyouth.org

Advocates for Youth is a nonprofit, nonpartisan organization dedicated to creating programs and promoting policies that help young people make informed and responsible decisions about their sexual health. It provides information, training, and advocacy to youth-serving organizations, policymakers, and the media in the United States and internationally. Depending on link or special area, the site is an excellent resource for teens and professionals. It has very current information and is updated frequently (at least monthly).

The site also provides good resources and materials for use and purchase, not only in English. The organization's specialized clearinghouses—on teen pregnancy prevention, HIV/STD prevention, school condom availability, peer education, school-based health centers, sexuality education, and adolescent reproductive health initiatives in developing countries—provide those developing and promoting programs and policies with critical, up-to-date information on relevant issues.

Some information is available in Spanish. "Di Que Si!" has sexuality information for teens in Spanish.

The site is very easy to use and has excellent links to other sites especially for teens, including transgender sites; gay, lesbian, and bisexual sites; international peer education sites; magazine sites; religious sexuality sites; safer sex sites; and youth-oriented sites. One site is designed by and for teens in Africa. This reviewer found that occasionally a link does not work as listed.

I wanna know.org: Answers to Your Questions About Teen Sexual Health and STD Prevention

http://www.iwannaknow.org

See review in Chapter 29, "Sexually Transmitted Diseases."

The Teen Pregnancy and Parenting Place

http://www.hometown.aol.com/mnn1121

See review in Chapter 27, "Pregnancy and Childbirth."

Teenshealth

http://www.teenshealth.org

This site is part of the larger "Kidshealth" Web site, sponsored by the Nemours Foundation. The Nemours Foundation was founded by philanthropist Alfred I. Dupont and is dedicated to improving the health of children and the elderly. Teenshealth is a colorful and attractive site addressing teen health issues. Sections include "Body Basics," "Mind Matters," "Sexual Health," food, fitness, and sports. At the time of this review there was a special feature on "How Can I Deal with My Anger?" The actual articles are readable accounts of teen peers managing the health problem being discussed, with practical tips on management and when to get help. Kidshealth has a large advisory board of medical professionals, who review the material on the site. The active TV-like appearance of the home page, and the first person accounts described in the articles should appeal to teens.

Chapter 4

Asthma and Allergies

Meg Smirnoff, MPH, RN, FNP and Kim Malusis, MS, RN, FNP

Allergies and asthma are sometimes merely annoying, at other times life threatening, and they are widespread. Despite improved understanding of the pathophysiology of asthma over the last 10 years, there has been a steady increase in the incidence and severity of the disease as reflected in morbidity, mortality, health care expenditures, and days lost to school or work. The understanding of asthma, which is often triggered by allergies, as an inflammatory process has revolutionized our treatment approach and added many highly effective agents to the therapeutic armamentarium. When used consistently, along with trigger control/avoidance, most cases of asthma can be controlled. Yet the current epidemic rates of asthma show that this scientific knowledge is not enough. Persons with asthma and their health care providers must find out how to use this knowledge. The following Web sites are good sources of information on asthma and allergies.

About.com: Asthma Section

http://asthma.about.com

This is a lively site that attempts to make easily accessible a wide range of information with a "common folks" approach. It is one of 700 under the larger About.com site. Each section is organized to offer a fully comprehensive "environment" around each topic, including up-to-date information, links with other Internet sites, how-to advice, and opportunities for questions and answers.

The site is directed at consumers and offers tie-ins to vendors of products that may interest them, such as makers of air purifiers. The advertisements are clearly marked and discrete from the consumer information. The information is comprehensive, current, and accurate.

The site has a broad range of topics, such as "Asthma Camp," "Back to School," and "Asthma-Friendly Sports," as well as standard information on support groups, triggers, and medications. Among the Web site tie-ins is an excellent site that focuses on pediatric asthma, *Kidshealth.about.cs.asthma.* Information is in English only. The site is fun, extremely interactive, easy to navigate, and very engaging.

American Academy of Allergy, Asthma, and Immunology

http://www.aaaai.org

This Web site is the public voice of the American Academy of Asthma, Allergy, and Immunology (AAAAI). Its purpose is to disseminate information about new research and technological advances, assist consumers in finding an allergist in their community, and provide public health education. Although the site represents the AAAAI, it is funded by Schering Plough Pharmaceutical Corp.

There is information specific for each group in the targeted audience. Consumers receive education, provider referrals in their community, and information on clinical trials being conducted all over the country from which they may benefit. Health care providers are offered professional resources, and the media are given an annotated, expanded explanation of new asthma/allergy technology. Any of the information may be used by the motivated consumer. The information is extremely current and accurate. The bulk of the information is in English only, although there is a listing of Spanish-language literature.

The AAAAI patient newsletter, *The Advocate*, is included in the Web site and can be downloaded. It has many interesting topics such as latex allergy, information on flu shots, managed care, and links between food reactions and behavior.

The site, which is written at a rather high level, may be daunting for some consumers and may require previous asthma knowledge. It is attractive and easy to navigate.

_____ Chapter **5**

Birth Control

Nancy E. Reame, PhD, RN, FAAN

_____

Information on birth control traditionally has been either hard to get or hard to ask about for teens and some adults. The Planned Parenthood site described below provides comprehensive information in the privacy and anonymity of the Internet.

Planned Parenthood

http://www.plannedparenthood.org

This Web site is sponsored by the Planned Parenthood Federation of America, Inc. (PPFA), the premier nonprofit advocacy organization for reproductive health care and birth control information/access. Established in 1916 by nurse Margaret Sanger, PPFA offers birth control information and reproductive health services with clinics across the country to women of all ages, regardless of their ability to pay.

The Web site offers a wide range of contraception information for both male and female consumers of all ages, as well as health professionals, in user-friendly language. The homepage is brightly colored and loaded with lots of interactive icons that transport the visitor to a large number of activities, services, and resources. Birth control methods are grouped into permanent (vasectomy for men, tubal sterilization for women) and temporary categories (e.g., abstinence, barrier, and hormonal methods). An important feature is the section on emergency contraception, which includes not only information on insertion of an intrauterine device after unprotected sex but also instructions for modifying standard doses of oral contraceptive for use as a "morning after" pill. To its credit, this Web site does more than just present the reproductive plumbing. Sections on the psychodynamics of contraception decision making, including how to negotiate condom use, permeate many of the pages devoted specifically to teens and preteens. However, once the visitor gets beyond the homepage, much of the substantive content is simple text rather than sophisticated graphics or visuals—perhaps an effort to distance itself from "adult" Web sites. Wisely, the homepage lists several links to other online resources on teen sexuality. Other features include press releases, a research section, a nurse practitioner program, greeting card messages, a search feature, and a store offering everything from PPFA coffee mugs to condom key chains. Teenwire.com, the winner of two Web site awards, is the interactive magazine tailored especially to teens and written in both English and Spanish. Because of the highly politicized nature of birth control and abortion in the United States, the emphasis on lobbying efforts and making donations to political action initiatives at the state, federal, and international levels may be a turn-off for antichoice visitors. Information on abortion services is included.

Additional Resource:
Not-2-Late.com: The Emergency Contraception Web Site

http://ec.princeton.edu

See review on page 18, in chapter on Medications.

Chapter 6

Breastfeeding

Kristen S. Montgomery, PhD, RNC, IBCLC

B reastfeeding offers significant advantages to both mothers and newborns and is recommended as the preferred infant feeding method by multiple professional organizations, including the American Academy of Pediatrics. Some of the more familiar benefits include a reduction in the number and severity of infections, particularly infant ear and respiratory infections. Additionally, breastfeeding offers significant advantages to mothers, including lower rates of certain types of reproductive cancers and more rapid postpartum weight loss. Despite these and other advantages, many women choose not to breastfeed or do not breastfeed beyond the early postpartum period.

A myriad of factors contribute to the low rates of breastfeeding initiation and duration that are currently prevalent in the United States. Two of the most significant factors include lack of information and lack of support. Many women do not receive adequate information regarding breastfeeding because of increasing distance between family members, lack of knowledge among family members who did not breastfeed their own children, low rates of breastfeeding in the most recent past (1970s), inadequate preparation of health care providers, and misleading or inappropriate information that is provided through vigorous infant formula marketing campaigns. Misunderstanding and lack of information contribute to environments in which women are not supported. The Web sites listed here can help to fill this gap and serve to educate and support women in their decision to breastfeed.

La Leche League International

http://www.lalecheleague.org

La Leche League International is one of the leading authorities on breastfeeding information, especially information for consumers. The purpose of the Web site is to provide a wide range of education and support to breastfeeding mothers. The site is sponsored by the organization, La Leche League International. The information that is provided in this site is current and accurate.

Some important features include a What's New section, news releases, information on finding support groups around the world, a section on frequently asked questions, an e-mail breastfeeding help form, where women can get answers from professionals (with an estimated time frame to receive an answer), online meetings (chat room), a section on breastfeeding and the law, a peer counselor program, and corporate lactation support. The site is available in English, Spanish, and Italian, and materials are available for order in a variety of languages. The information provided is high level. The Web site is aesthetically pleasing and easy to navigate.

Medela

http://www.medela.com

This site allows breastfeeding women and health care professionals to access information related to the art and science of breastfeeding. It provides support and information on breastfeeding. Included is a description of feeding techniques, treatments for common feeding problems, available feeding equipment, and a variety of links to access breastfeeding professionals. Medela.com is intended for laypeople, particularly nursing mothers, as well as health professionals who are involved in the care of breastfeeding women.

The sponsor is Medela International, a manufacturer of breastfeeding products, including breast pumps. La Leche League International, a grassroots self-help support organization, is a supporter of the Web site (see separate entry).

The site provides accurate, current, carefully worded information that is easy to read and understand.

REVIEWED BY JANE WEISER, EDD, RN, IBCLC

Nanny's Place: Breastfeeding

http://www.moonlily.com/breastfeed

Nanny's Place: Breastfeeding is a support and information site for breastfeeding mothers and their families. The site is copyrighted and maintained by Donna Zelzer, a mother, grandmother, and writer. It is intended for families, mothers, mothers-to-be, and women considering pregnancy. The information provided is current and accurate. One of the best features of this site is the information that is provided in brief articles. The site also provides personal stories and examples that are likely to be helpful to breastfeeding mothers and those considering breastfeeding. Resources are provided for consumers to purchase products and find additional information. The site author also offers a newsletter to those individuals who provide an e-mail address for this purpose. This site is part of a larger network of maternity and child care information.

The site currently is not available in any other languages. The information is provided at a high level. The site is well organized, easy to use, and colorful.

The Nursing Lounge

http://www.parentingweb.com/lounge/lounge_index.htm

The Nursing Lounge is one section of a large parenting site. The purpose of this site is to provide information and interaction for nurturing parents. The Parenting Web (*parentingweb.com*) and Keri Baker produce the site. Consumers are the site's intended audience. The information provided is accurate and current. The site features several significant advantages. Both basic and more advanced topics are included, and there are sections on breastfeeding myths, problems, and solutions, as well as specific breastfeeding situations. There is also a list of feature articles that cover a variety of topics.

Information is provided only in English, although the site is very easy to use and features calming colors for potentially frantic new parents. The information is average to high level and presented in a concise and clear format.

ProMoM: Promotion of Mother's Milk Inc.

http://promom.org

Promotion of Mother's Milk, Inc. identifies the organization as: "a non-profit dedicated to increasing public awareness and public acceptance of breastfeeding." The information provided throughout the site is accurate and current. Some of the more important features include articles and essays by leading breastfeeding authorities, and a section on 101 reasons to breastfeed your child. There are also links to other resources, a library, products, and professionals. Message boards, chat rooms, mailing lists, and committees are additional highlights of the site. Additionally, the site has a professional advisory board, information on breastfeeding myths, and a list of breastfeeding-friendly physicians, hospitals, and businesses.

The site is not currently available in any other language. The content is presented at an average level. The site is easy to use.

_____ Chapter 7

Cancer

Françoise Juste, BSN, RNC and Trudy Johnson, MA, RN, CNAA

The Internet sites reviewed in this chapter originate mainly from various professional organizations and government agencies whose primary mission is to provide current information on different types of cancer, treatment options, clinical trials, support systems, and fact sheets for patients and family members.

There are numerous cancer-related sites available. The sites reviewed here focused primarily on how and where to obtain support services, how to make informed decisions regarding treatment options, and how to gather or use information on a specific topic.

American Cancer Society

http://www.cancer.org

The American Cancer Society is a large nonprofit health care organization, specifically designed to aid the community. The organization's mission is to eliminate cancer as a major health issue through prevention, research, education, advocacy, and service. The link "Cancer Resource Center" offers answers to questions about the nature, causes, and risk factors of cancer. A special feature of this site is the link "Cancer Survivor Network," which gives support to cancer survivors. Consumers may obtain free brochures and leaflets in English and Spanish.

The site design is user-friendly, allowing consumers to obtain the latest version of guidelines on different types of cancer. The links, graphics, and text are easy to navigate and readable. The information is current and maintained routinely.

A disclaimer describing the limitations, scope, timeliness of posting, and source of information is given. The disclaimer includes a statement that the content is to be used for general health information and does not indicate medical advice.

Overall, this site is consistent, clear, and concise. Consumers will obtain comprehensive information covering cancer research, treatment, and education. The reading level of the site probably requires at least a high school education.

American Society of Clinical Oncology

http://www.asco.org

The nonprofit American Society of Clinical Oncology (ASCO) represents more than 15,000 cancer professionals and members worldwide. The organization was founded in 1964 by a group of physicians from the American Association of Cancer Research. This site supports all types of cancer research, in particular, patient-oriented clinical research.

The drop-down menu has a feature titled "People Living with Cancer" that offers the consumer many choices, from finding an oncologist in any given region to participating in clinical trials. The ASCO "Media Center" link provides information on news releases, annual meetings, and public policy. User also may review the *Journal of Clinical Oncology* online.

There are numerous useful and educational tools available for cancer patients and their significant others on this site:

1. Patient guides are available on advanced lung cancer treatment, treatment for breast cancer, prevention and treatment of nausea and vomiting caused by chemotherapy, and follow-up care for colorectal cancer.
2. A search engine database can be used to locate an oncologist in any given region.
3. A glossary offers definitions of terms.
4. A search function is available using keywords for types of cancer and category. Users can search the site by targeting a particular

type of cancer or selecting a category that reflects a specific choice or interest. Currently, information is available for four major types of cancer: breast, lung, prostate, and colon.
5. A comprehensive list of recommended hyperlinks is available for consumers and professionals.

The ASCO site serves as a valuable resource for consumers and professionals seeking credible information on current news on cancer. The "Cancer in the News" feature offers cancer patients and their families current information they need to assess and evaluate what they hear or read about cancer. The ongoing roster titled "This week on ASCO Online" gives a quick overview of the features for the week. The site is easy to navigate, easy to use, and well organized. The education level required is high school.

Cancer Care

http://www.cancercare.org

Cancer Care, Inc. is a nonprofit national organization whose mission is to assist people with cancer through support, counseling, and appropriate referral. Services are available to people of all ages, with all types of cancer, and at any stage of the disease. In addition to patients, the intended audience includes professionals, family members, and caregivers. To facilitate access for the Spanish-speaking population, the content is also available in Spanish.

Cancer Care Inc. has a list of all the organizations and companies that helped sponsor this site by providing various related information. Links to professional sites are available, including the American Society of Clinical Oncology, the Oncology Nursing Society, and the National Cancer Institute.

The "Helping Hand Resource Guide" is a search function for local and national agencies that help people with cancer. Teleconferences are also a vital service of the organization, and these are posted on the site.

The design is efficient and easy to follow. The information is geared for persons with a least some high school education. However, the resource and counseling information would be useful for a lower educational level.

Cancer Education

http://www.cancereducation.com

The mission of this site is "to improve cancer care through the dissemination of up-to-date and accurate educational programming and information for health care professionals, cancer patients and their family members." This site is divided into two categories, the "Patient and Family Center" and the "Professional Center." For the purposes of this book, the review will focus on the former.

The "Patient and Family Center" has a drop-down menu listing all types of cancer. As the consumer enters the type of cancer selected, a jump screen appears with all the appropriate links pertinent to the selection of the cancer type. The focus of the site is uniquely to educate patients with high-quality online resources and tools. The site makes it easy for the consumer to obtain information on an abundance of topics, including coverage of over 20 types of cancer, *Merriam Webster's Collegiate Dictionary* for term definition, and physician and cancer treatment center directories. In addition, the site offers a message board designed for professionals, patients, or family members to post various questions to be answered in a forum format. The site design is user-friendly, easy to navigate, and readable by educated persons. The links are easily accessible and serve as a useful guide to the consumer.

Cancereducation.com is funded primarily by specific charitable groups and organizations, including Adelphi New York Statewide Breast Cancer Hotline and Support Program, CancerCare, Inc., Cure for Lymphoma Foundation, Inc., International Myeloma Foundation, Multiple Myeloma Research Foundation, WAR (Women at Risk), the Brain Tumor Society, the Kidney Cancer Association, the Leukemia Society of America (New York City chapter), and the Wellness Community of Philadelphia.

The site is for the "savvy consumer" and is targeted to consumers with some college education.

Cancerfacts

http://www.cancerfacts.com

Cancerfacts is operated by Nexcura, Inc., a leading e-care company that develops Web-based applications for physicians, patients, and family members. These applications are geared to making the appropriate decision to achieve an optimal goal and care outcome. The target audiences are physicians and consumers.

The site is dedicated to providing accurate, meaningful, and comprehensive information to help people make informed decisions about cancer. Cancerfacts has a shared partnership with Medical Economics Co., publisher and developer of the *Physician Desk Reference* (PDR).

One unique, exciting, and innovative feature of this site is "The Cancer Profiler" interactive online tool. It is designed as a decision tool to help patients make crucial decisions about treatment options. This is an extremely valuable tool that allows consumers to assimilate the extensive information available about treatment options for cancer. Additionally, "The Cancer Profiler" takes into consideration variables, such as quality of life, that may essentially affect one's treatment decision. The site also assures the user that all personal information is kept confidential and secure. A powerful encryption program by VeriSign protects and guards the data.

The screen design is simple, straightforward, and businesslike. There is no use of extra graphics or pictures. The links are very easy to find and serve as a useful guide to the consumer. The site is recommended for individuals who are looking to maximize their quality of life and outcomes by making the right educational decisions about treatment options.

Cancernet

http://www.cancernet.nci.nih.gov

Cancernet is a service from the National Cancer Institute (NCI), the principal agency of the federal government for cancer research. NCI is a main component of the National Institutes of Health that provides current, comprehensible, and credible information on cancer. The purpose of this site is to make information readily accessible for the consumer regarding types of cancer, treatment options, clinical trials, support services, testing, prevention genetics, coping with cancer, and cancer literature.

Cancernet's information is considered reliable and valid because it is derived from the Physician Data Query, the National Cancer Institutes Database. The information is revised and updated by experts in oncology and related cancer specialties. The material on the site has current information published within one week of the author's review.

The intended audience is anyone with a question on cancer, in particular patients and their families and friends, as well as health care professionals and caregivers. Unique to this site is the ability of the user to select links that address other specific cancer topics of interests, including genetic risk for cancer. Links are considered reliable because the site has a published policy stating that the links must be consistent with the Cancernet mission and are subject to adequate process review.

Overall, the site's design is very conservative in its presentation and is easy to follow and read. The site has a user-friendly site map to help the first-time visitor maneuver around the site and search the topic of interest.

Oncolink

http://www.oncolink.com

Cancer specialists at the University of Pennsylvania Cancer Center (UPCC) founded this site to provide free information related to cancer for patients, families, and health care professionals. Comprehensive resources are available from this site for consumers and professionals. The topics include updates on specific types of cancer treatment and news about advances in research. The menus are user-friendly, particularly for persons who do not use the Internet frequently.

The disease-oriented menus are comprehensive. The most valuable feature is the searchable database about clinical trials at the UPCC. The section "Cutting Edge Research" highlights emerging technologies and approaches to cancer care that are not yet available for treatment.

The *Cancer News* links to recently published press articles summarizing scholarly findings in understandable terms. For the professional there is a "Conferences and Meetings" section, which includes not only conferences at UPCC but also national conferences that are submitted to Oncolink for publishing on the site. The "Book Reviews" section provides summaries of books on cancer with a link to *Amazon.com* if the user wants to make a purchase at the same time.

Chapter 8

Child Health

Wendy M. Nehring, PhD, RN, Sandra A. Faux, PhD, RN, and Cynthia A. Schmidt, PhD, RN

The health of children encompasses not only illness care but also health promotion. A safe, secure, and wholesome environment, with adequate nutritional intake, physical activity, and educational opportunities, is of primary concern. The Web sites listed here take this comprehensive approach to children's health.

Children's Defense Fund

http://www.childrensdefense.org

This site has been designed to inform consumers and professionals about program and policy issues related to the well-being of children in the United States. Ongoing projects, research, and current statistics are available, particularly health information related to uninsured children, maternal and child health, immunizations, and Medicaid. The types of information includes descriptions of successful outreach and enrollment strategies, national and state data, proposed and adopted federal and state legislation, and developments in state and local child health policy.

The mission of the Children's Defense Fund (CDF) is to "Leave no child behind and to ensure every child a healthy start, a head start, a fair start, a safe start, and a moral start in life and successful passage to adulthood with the help of caring families and communities." It is a voice for children, particularly the poor, minority, and disabled. The CDF is a private, nonprofit organization supported by foundations, corporation grants, and individual donations.

The site is aimed at primarily adult consumers who are seeking information about issues affecting the children noted above. However, it is also very useful for health care professionals seeking current policy information and statistics about children (e.g., gun violence and uninsured statistics).

It is my opinion that the information presented on this Web site is current and accurate. The site's strongest points are the currency of the information and the archived information. The site is also well organized and easily navigable. Many consumers may be turned off by the complexity of the information (e.g., statistical reports), and to read some materials the user has to have Adobe Acrobat, which may provide a barrier for some users. The site is available only in English. Overall, both lay and professional consumers will find this to be a useful and informative site concerning children and their health and development.

SANDRA A. FAUX, PHD, RN

Health and Human Services Pages for Kids

http://www.hhs.gov/kids

This site provides links to Web pages designed specifically for children on topics related to child health from several leading federal agencies, such as the National Cancer Institute and the National Clearinghouse for Alcohol and Drug Information. The purpose of this site is to provide links from federal agencies on topics related to child health that would be creative and presented at a level appropriate for children. The site is produced by the Department of Health and Human Services.

The site's intended audience is children. Several of the links, including the homepage, have information for parents, teachers, and/or health professionals on additional information related to the topic and suggestions for class and/or clinical presentation. A "kid's privacy" notice is also included on the homepage.

The information presented is current and accurate. In general, the best feature of this site is the diversity of links presented to children on child health topics. Examples include smoke-free kids and soccer, crime, global health, and hazardous waste sites and children's health risks. Although not a weakness, some of the links are more creatively presented than others. The majority of information on this site is in English. Only a few links provide content in both English and Spanish. The level of the information presented in this site is average. Each link is presented at an age-appropriate level for school-aged children. Information for parents, teachers, and health professionals is also at a level appropriate for the average audience. The site is an excellent source of links on child health care–related topics.

WENDY M. NEHRING, PHD, RN

National Center for Education in Maternal and Child Health

http://www.ncemch.org

This site provides comprehensive information on national child health policy, projects, and programmatic policy information. Emphasis is placed on Bright Futures, the Healthy Start National Resource Center, the National Maternal and Child Health Clearinghouse, and current national guidelines, conference proceedings, and relevant publications.

The purpose of this site is to present up-to-date national information on current child health topics, policy analysis and education, and program development to improve the health and well-being of this country's children and their families. The site is produced by Georgetown University's Public Policy Institute and is supported by the Maternal and Child Health Bureau, a part of the Health Resources and Services Administration. The intended audiences are health care professionals and lay consumers.

The information presented is current, accurate, and state of the art. The best feature of this site is the availability of publications either on this site or in printed form. The publications are sorted by categories, such as child care, children's health insurance, health supervision, infant mortality, and racial and ethnic disparities. The publications include guidelines for practice, factual support for child health policy, and research results. The information on the site is available only in English; however, most of the publications can be ordered in Spanish. The level of the information presented in this site is high. Technical language is used.

The site is an excellent source of comprehensive information on the full range of current child health topics.

WENDY M. NEHRING, PHD, RN

National Institute of Child Health and Human Development

http://www.nichd.nih.gov

This site provides comprehensive information on child health and the media, research resources, and epidemiology, statistics, and prevention. The category of child health information and the media includes publications, current news releases, information specialists, and national campaigns. The purpose of this site is to present current national information on child health and developmental topics. The site is produced by the National Institute of Child Health and Human Development, an agency under the National Institutes of Health. The intended audiences are health care professionals and lay consumers.

The majority of information presented is current, accurate, and state of the art. A few of the publications, however, are more than five years old. In general, the best features of this site are the available publications, resource list of information specialists, and press releases on current topics. Most of the publications are reports of proceedings or health information. A weak point is that all publications are not free and downloadable. The information on this site is available only in English.

This site is an excellent source of comprehensive information on a variety of child health care–related topics and current statistics on the status of child health in the United States.

WENDY M. NEHRING, PHD, RN

National Resource Center for Health and Safety in Child Care

http://nrc.uchsc.edu

This site provides comprehensive national information on health and safety performance standards, individual state child care licensure regulations, the full text of "Stepping Stones to Using Caring for Our

Children," links to other child care information resources, and health and safety tips. The purpose of this site is to present information to "promote health and safety in out-of-home child care settings throughout the nation." The site is produced by the National Resource Center for Health and Safety in Child Care at the University of Colorado Health Science Center, School of Nursing, and is funded by the U.S. Maternal and Child Health Bureau. The intended audiences are health care professionals and lay consumers.

The information presented is current, accurate, and state of the art. The best features are the current child care licensure regulations for each state in the United States and Washington, DC, and the "National Health and Safety Performance Standards Guidelines for Out-of-Home Child Care Programs." The information is available only in English. Technical language is used. The site is an excellent source of comprehensive information on the current state of child health and safety in the United States.

WENDY M. NEHRING, PHD, RN

World Health Organization, Division of Child Health and Development

http://www.who.int/chd

The site provides visitors with extensive information regarding the efforts of the World Health Organization's (WHO) Division of Child Health and Development (CHD). Its purpose is to provide guidelines, updates of progress, and research information to health professionals and provide up-to-date information to the media. The site is sponsored by the WHO but can be reached only after multiple clicks from that organization's homepage. Visitors should go directly to the site address listed above.

The intended audience includes health professionals, members of the press, and any other individuals interested in the health of the world's children and the efforts being taken "to decrease the mortality and morbidity and to promote health, growth and development for all children."

Information provided is inclusive of research dating to the early 1980s, yet it also includes some recent publications. Guidelines provided for practitioners are the latest recommendations, are detailed, and provide adaptations for various countries.

From the homepage of CHD, visitors can click to seven different sites. The first is "Integrated Management of Childhood Illness (IMCI)," which offers extensive information about the efforts to manage the conditions that cause 7 of 10 childhood deaths. Reports from recent worldwide meetings, research literature, guidelines for treatment and prevention, and current statistics are available. Three additional sites, "Acute Respiratory Infections (ARI)," "Diarrheal Diseases (CDD)," and "Cholera," offer basic facts, management guidelines, and reference lists dealing with each of the respective topics. The three remaining sites, "Documents," "Links," and "Search," offer more direct access to requested information and documentation.

Information is given in English, French, and Spanish. The level of information provided is high, and information for the media was appropriate.

CYNTHIA A. SCHMIDT, PHD, RN

Chapter 9

Complementary and Alternative Therapies

Mariah Snyder, PhD, RN, FAAN

The number of Web sites for complementary therapies is growing as rapidly as the field of complementary/alternative therapies. It is incumbent on health professionals to become knowledgeable about sites that are relevant to therapies they administer because consumers will be accessing these sites and may question health professionals about the content noted on each site. The quality of content included on the sites varies. Three sites are reviewed: a comprehensive site on complementary therapies and two relating to specific therapies.

American Botanical Council

http://www.herbalgram.org

This is the Web site for the American Botanical Council, which is a nonprofit research and education organization. The site has a predominantly commercial focus, with selling educational products related to herbal preparation as its main focus. It is a vehicle for the American Botanical Council, whose mission is "to provide services which further the dissemination of responsible, science-based information on herbs and phytomedicines." The site provides information on many books and monographs on herbal preparations. Additionally, it presents press releases that describe findings from studies on herbal preparations. Links with other sites are provided.

45

The format of this site may be misleading to users. For example, education on the menu brings users in touch with publications and not specific information about a specific herbal preparation. The site does present current information about publications and press releases about research. It also provides information on funding agencies for specific projects.

National Center for Complementary and Alternative Medicine

http://www.nccam.nih.gov

This is the Web site for the Center for Complementary/Alternative Medicine (NCCAM) at the National Institutes of Health. It is a multipurpose site that provides information for health professionals and consumers. The site contains general information about NCCAM and the programs and services it offers, as well as an overview of complementary therapies. A number of features of the site would be of interest to consumers: general information on assessing the safety and effectiveness of a therapy, selecting a practitioner, and determining how complementary/alternative therapies are integrated into health care. In addition to general information about complementary/alternative medicine (CAM), directions for accessing other sites for additional information are provided. These include *http://chid.nih.gov* (alternative medicine category on the Combined Health Information Database), on which persons can access abstracts of articles and books. The telephone numbers for various services of NCCAM are provided. Of particular interest to consumers is the NCCAM Clearinghouse; information from the clearinghouse is available in both English and Spanish. The main menu also provides access to the organization's quarterly newsletter from which the latest information on a number of therapies is available.

This site is easy to use, and the menu is easy to follow. The site contains an extensive amount of information and provides access to other sources of information about complementary/alternative medicine. It is updated on a regular basis. One feature that is not included is access to various professional organizations related to the subject. These are most likely not included because, as NCCAM clearly notes, the organization is not a referral agency for complementary/alternative therapies or for practitioners.

Precious Aromatherapy

http://www.aromatherapy.com

This is the Web site for Precious Aromatherapy, a commercial firm. The site offers extensive information on aromatherapy, including a description of aromatherapy and essential oils and a review of many essential oils, including their botanical and common names. Although the site would appear to be aimed at health professionals or others using essential oils, consumers would find the content informative. A precautionary note is found at the beginning of the description of essential oils, stating that "modern medical research has not been conducted to confirm or disprove the effectiveness of essential oils." An extensive list of books on aromatherapy is given. Resources for obtaining education on aromatherapy is provided. Because this is a commercial site, the opportunity to purchase essential oils is available.

The site is easy to use, and the menu is easy to follow. The amount of information contained on the site is amazing. The information appears to be current.

Chapter 10

Diabetes Mellitus

Rita G. Mertig, MS, RNC, CNS

Individuals with diabetes mellitus have many questions about living with this chronic condition that affects every aspect of their lives. Many seek this information on the World Wide Web. The following sites have been explored for content, usability, and up-to-date information about the many aspects of the management of diabetes as well as current and future developments that may enhance life with diabetes. Because there are many other sites that deal with diabetes, the following guidelines should be useful in personally evaluating these other sites for current and accurate information. The American Diabetes Association made the following recommendations at its Summer 1997 convention. Use them to help judge whether or not the site you are looking at is up-to-date.

1. Be sure that the site uses the most current terminology for type 1 diabetes (formerly called insulin-dependent or juvenile diabetes) and type 2 diabetes (formerly called non-insulin-dependent or adult onset diabetes). Type 1 can be first diagnosed in adults well into their 60s. Type 2 diabetes is being diagnosed in overweight teenagers, and many patients with type 2 diabetes must use insulin to control blood sugars.
2. If the site lists the diagnostic criteria for diabetes, it should use a fasting blood sugar of 126 mg/dL, not the older 140 mg/dL. The site also should list the current recommendations for testing the adult population, which include:

   - All adults should be given a fasting blood sugar at 45 years of age and every 3 years thereafter.

- Those who are African-American, Native American, Hispanic, or Asian and/or who have a family history of diabetes, are overweight, and have hypertension or hyperlipidemia should be tested at an earlier age and at more frequent intervals.

3. In addition, you should note if the authors of the site are attempting to sell a product from which they will gain financially. This does not necessarily invalidate the information presented, but it does make it biased.
4. If investigating a chat room designed for children, their parents, or adults with diabetes, look for a knowledgeable person who monitors the site for misinformation. Be sure to present the information that you get from these sites to your physician or diabetes educator for validation.

American Diabetes Association

http://www.diabetes.org

This site is the most comprehensive, informative, accurate, and current of all the sites examined. The American Diabetes Association (ADA) is responsible for the content of this site and as such ensures that the information is reliable and current. The site is designed primarily for patients, their families, and anyone interested in learning about diabetes. It also has a section for health professionals and practitioners looking for the latest research and care guidelines for managing patients with Type 1 or Type 2 diabetes. Users can download articles from *Diabetes Forecast*, a journal written for people with diabetes and their family members, as well as the organization's five professional journals. Because of the inclusion of these articles, the site has well over 10,000 pages, more than any other diabetes-related Web site.

The site is colorful and inviting, is easy to use, and has many links to a wide variety of topics, such as diabetes in the news, diabetes management guidelines, information on weight loss and nutrition, glycemic index, eating out, recipes, exercise, medication, advocacy, insurance needs, work-related items, children with diabetes, and sports figures and celebrities with diabetes. All of the articles are written for consumers in simple, easy-to-understand language. The links provide practical advice in a positive and upbeat manner. Links to other health organizations make looking for related topics such as kidney disease, hypertension, and cardiovascular disease easy. The ADA can be sent e-mail by clicking on "E-mail Us" at the bottom of the left-hand column after the organization's phone number. The largest section on diabetes information is also available in Spanish.

Children with Diabetes

http://www.childrenwithdiabetes.com

This site is maintained jointly by Children with Diabetes, whose mission is to promote understanding of the care and treatment of diabetes, especially in children, and Diabetes 123, whose mission is to be the world leader in online diabetes care, improving the quality and reducing the cost of care, and Diabetes Monitor, which is dedicated to helping persons with diabetes to educate themselves about their role as active participants in the care of this disorder. The authors of this informative Web site describe it as "the on-line community for kids, families and adults with diabetes." It includes recipes and chat rooms, as well as accurate and timely information events, conferences, research, and other news concerning living with diabetes. The site conducts polls, answers frequently asked questions, maintains a link to diabetes-related product sites, and offers tips on helping children with diabetes. *Children with Diabetes* subscribes to the HONcode principles of the Health On the Net Foundation.

The Diabetes Mall

http://www.diabetesnet.com

This is the site of The Diabetes Mall and is described by the company as the "leading Web-based source of information and retail products focused exclusively on diabetes." The authors of this site further describe their services as providing "the Web's most comprehensive weekly online diabetes newspaper, *Diabetes This Week*, plus research reports, articles analyzing current diabetes issues, interactive tools for better blood sugar control, contests and information on the latest drugs, medications, devices, products, diets, blood sugar management tools and future developments in diabetes care." The online store at this site "offers the widest array of competitively priced diabetes books, software, scales, and other products to educate, entertain, and inform."

Directors John Walsh and Ruth Roberts founded The Diabetes Mall in 1994. They have personal and professional knowledge of diabetes and have written extensively on the subject. The authors describe the Mall's competitive edge as "living in the same world as our customers. All of our current staff (at the Mall) either have diabetes or have a close family member with it." The Diabetes Mall offers 20% to 25% discounts on books, software, and many other diabetes products. These products are described in detail. Ordering is very simple, and the site is secure for giving credit card information. The Mall's e-mail address is *webmaster@diabetesnet.com*, or orders can be placed by phone at (800-988-4772).

Other departments that can be accessed through this site include research, fun sites, control tips, diabetes information, Internet resources, the latest technology, alternative therapies, and complications. Each of these includes multiple links to a variety of information, or you can use the search tool and indicate your desire for "verbose" or "simple" information, with a maximum number of results to be inserted. There is even a site that will figure out insulin needs for Type 1 diabetics based on weight and activity level. The site is very entertaining and easy to use.

Insulin Pumpers

http://www.insulin-pumpers.org

This site provides information and support for adults and children with diabetes and their families who are interested in insulin pump therapy. It belongs to the members of the Insulin Pumpers Organization and, as such, is not promoting any specific manufacturer's products. Links include information on the organization; chat rooms; a search engine for information on diabetes and insulin pump sites; questions and answers on diabetes and insulin pumps; a how-to section concerning the use of insulin pumps, carbo counting, snacks, and recipes; and a physician referral directory. This very informative and helpful site is subsidized in part by Animas, Disetronics, and MiniMed, manufacturers of insulin pumps, as well as contributions from members. The organization subscribes to the HONcode principles of the Health On the Net Foundation. The e-mail address is *Editor@Insulin-Pumpers.org*.

Joslin Diabetes Center

http://www.joslin.org

This informative and authoritative site is published by the Joslin Diabetes Center of Boston, which is affiliated with the Harvard Medical School. The purpose of the site is to educate patients and professionals on the various aspects of diabetes, with up-to-date information on research and new developments in the field of diabetes.

The site is easy to navigate and to understand, with multiple links to diabetes in the news, diabetes management, and professional education. The research tends to be mostly that which is being done at the Joslin Diabetes Center, and the lack of dates for this research makes it difficult to judge how current the information is.

There are discussion boards where questions can be asked of the experts, and questions can be e-mailed to *diabetes@joslin.harvard.edu*. There also are help links for those who are new to the Internet.

Juvenile Diabetes Foundation International
The Diabetes Research Foundation

http://www.jdf.org

The Juvenile Diabetes Foundation International (JDF) maintains this site. JDF was founded in 1970 by parents of children with diabetes with the mission of finding a cure for diabetes and its complications through support of research. As such, it is primarily a nonprofit diabetes research foundation interested in diabetes in children in general, and Type 1 diabetes in particular. The information is intended for the parents of children with diabetes, their children, and anyone who deals with children with diabetes, such as teachers and babysitters.

The site has useful and accurate information and is presented in a user-friendly way. There are specific sections for school-aged children, preadolescents, and teenagers to help them in an age-appropriate manner to understand and manage their health. Links to other sites of interest to children and their parents are also represented. There is even a JDF Kids online policy to help parents evaluate sites in which their children might be interested. A Q&A section answers many common questions asked and specific questions can be e-mailed to *info@jdfcure.org*. Links have pictures of active, healthy children and deliver positive, easy-to-relate-to messages for parents. Medical terms used are defined.

The one drawback is that most of the material is written at a high level, which may be difficult to comprehend for some parents and most children. There is, however, a list of books for children at various ages, which look to be age appropriate. These books can be ordered from the Juvenile Diabetes Foundation. Most of the material is from *Countdown* magazine, which is published by JDF.

Rick Mendosa's Diabetes Directory

http://www.mendosa.com/diabetes.htm

This is the site of *Rick Mendosa's Diabetes Dictionary*. Mendosa, a freelance journalist and consultant, specializes in articles on diabetes care. He also has Type 2 diabetes. He researches and writes reports for various magazines, newsletters, medical/technical companies, and professional organizations, including the American Diabetes Association (ADA). Mendosa is known and is respected as an in-depth writer and is described by the ADA as someone with "absolute journalistic objectivity." His site also can be accessed through the site maintained by the American Diabetes Association (see separate entry) at *http://www.diabetes.org/mendosa*.

Mendosa frequently updates the site with his latest columns concerning diabetes and related matters and offers numerous links to his other well-researched articles. He has maintained this site since 1995. Categories under which he lists Internet links include online diabetes resources, which includes frequently asked questions, diabetes-related organizations and charities, companies and institutions that deal with diabetes-related information, products and research, diabetes-related publications, government Web sites, diabetes software, Medline resources dealing with diabetes, and a site with current information on diabetes medication, including insulin, blood glucose meters, and long-term diabetes complications. There are also links to articles written for *NutriNews.com* and for *DiabetesWebSite.com*, as well as freebies and rebates. The Web site is easy to use, informative, and well worth the time for anyone interested in exploring diabetes. Rick Mendosa's e-mail address is *mendosa@mendosa.com*.

Chapter 11

Diet, Nutrition, and Weight Loss

Karen H. Morin, DSN, RN

T his chapter presents information related to diet, nutrition, and weight loss. Although an attempt was made to separate the two topics, many Web sites, including the ones presented here, discuss one or all of the topics under most of the sites. Most sites have a history on the Internet and are user-friendly; thus, you do not need to be a computer expert to navigate the sites. All sites are relevant to health care professionals as well as consumers. Only one site provides information in Spanish.

American Dietetic Association

http://www.eatright.org

This Web site is the homepage for the American Dietetic Association. Accessing the site map provides information on what is available for consumers and health care providers. Users can obtain information on nutrition and healthy lifestyles (including weight loss). In addition, there are resources listed separately for consumers and professionals, with links for easy access.

Although rather linear in presentation, this site is easy to navigate. Information, available only in English, is accurate, current, and not difficult to understand.

Foodfit.com

http://www.foodfit.com

This is a commercial site that was founded by consumer advocate Ellen Haas (former undersecretary for Food, Nutrition, and Consumer Services at the U.S. Department of Agriculture) to help consumers lead healthier lives. Information on nutrition and fitness is easily accessed through visually appealing icons on the homepage. Recipes, nutritional information, and tips on fitness are available. In addition, users may choose to become members of Foodfit and avail themselves of more personal information.

Foodfit has an advisory board that is comprised of, but not limited to, physicians with expertise in nutrition, restaurant owners, and chefs. Information is accurate and very timely. The level of information is average. Most users should not have difficulty understanding the information presented.

The site is visually appealing, seasonal in nature, and easy to interpret. The organization of information invites users to explore what is available.

New York Online Access to Health

http://www.noah-health.org

NOAH (New York Online Access to Health) provides "high-quality full-text health information for consumers that is accurate, timely, relevant and unbiased." (See review of site in Chapter 1.)

Its nutrition pages address the broad topics of "General Information," "Nutrition and Aging," "Nutrition and Pregnancy," "Nutrition and Disease," "Food Biotechnology/Radiation," and "Nutrition and Children." Each topic is divided into categories that are extensive in nature. Information about when each category was updated is provided in the overview.

Information presented is accurate and timely. Overall, the site is user-friendly.

Nutrition Navigator: A Rating Guide to Nutrition Web Sites

http://www.navigator.tufts.edu

This site is invaluable in directing health care providers and consumers to additional sites that have been rated using criteria developed by nutrition specialists in Canada and the United States. It was developed to address two specific concerns Web users have when seeking information: (1) quick access and (2) trustworthy information. The Web site is maintained by Tufts University School of Nutrition Science and Policy. Rated sites are categorized by broad topics, such as "General Nutrition," "Kids," and "Health Professionals." Information on each site is rated for currency. This site is visually appealing, simple in design, and very user-friendly. The hyperlinks to other sites enhance access of information. To date, information is available in English only. The level of information is considered high level, in that each site listed has been evaluated using well-articulated criteria.

Weight-Control Information Network

http://www.niddk.nih.gov/health/nutrit/win.htm

The Weight-Control Information Network (WIN) site provides data-based information to health care providers and to consumers on obesity, weight control, and nutrition. The National Institute of Diabetes and Digestive and Kidney Disease (NIDDK) of the National Institutes of Health is responsible for its oversight. This site provides links to publications, to programs sponsored by NIDDK, and to clinical nutrition research centers and units. In addition, a link to the Combined Health Information Database (CHID) is included. This link provides access to an extensive reference list of books, articles, and educational materials on obesity and weight loss. The site is easy to access, with little to distract the user from the task at hand: obtaining accurate information about obesity and weight loss.

Currently, the site is in English only. A nice feature of this site is the inclusion of the pilot campaign encouraging weight control in African-American women in the Boston area. The level of information is simple. This site is invaluable for persons interested in obesity and weight loss.

Chapter 12

Domestic Violence and Child Abuse

Jacquelyn C. Campbell, PhD, RN, FAAN, Dorothy Lemmey, PhD, RN, and Kathryn Chouaf, MSN, RN

A national random survey estimated that 4.4 million adult women are abused by a significant other every year in the U.S. (Plichta, 1997). Studies have found varying rates of abuse in diverse departments of the health care system. In the emergency department, 68% reported being assaulted by their current partner (Hotch, Grunfeld, Mackay, & Cowan, 1996); in pediatric settings, 10% were assaulted by a current partner (Duffy, McGrath, Becker, & Linakis, 1999); and during pregnancy, approximately 4–8% were assaulted (Gazmararian et al., 1996).

Universal screening in health care settings of all women is strongly recommended. When abuse is found, health professionals need excellent and varied resources to guide their interventions; these Web sites can be an invaluable resource for women. They are easily accessible at home or libraries, and less likely to be detected by an abusive mate than printed literature. If the home PC is used, they must clear their cache just before closing the web browser to prevent an abusive partner from discovering the web sites visited (directions to clear cache can be found at *http://dotlemmey.freeyellow.com/clear_your_cache.htm*). For more complete information to assist battered women and their children refer to Campbell (1998).

American Bar Association Against Domestic Violence

http://www.abanet.org/domviol/home.html

This web site is primarily for legal assistance to victims' attorneys and victims of domestic violence. The stated objective is to develop a comprehensive, multidisciplinary blueprint for communities seeking effective responses to domestic violence. The site is sponsored by the American Bar Association, specifically, the Commission on Domestic Violence, which is made up of legal, judicial, and medical professionals.

The intended audience is primarily legal advocates and organizations assisting victims. It was chosen because of the link to multistate pro bono organizations for survivors, as well as state bar associations to contact for free legal services in specific states. The site does not indicate updates. Therefore, it is difficult to determine when it was last updated.

The most important feature of this site is its interactive methods for obtaining a listing of pro bono services, searchable by state. There is also a lawyer referral service for specific states, for those who cannot afford a lawyer. It also has a search engine for researching domestic violence. It is not directed to an under-8th grade educated reader. There is no multilingual support. The overall level of this information is directed toward more highly educated individuals, but there are easy to understand links for survivors such as 5 ways to fight domestic violence, which informs them of their rights and provides a safety plan. The ease of use to access legal services is its strength for survivors.

Family Peace Project: Medical College of Wisconsin

http://www.family.mcw.edu/FamilyPeaceProject.htm

The Family Peace Project site provides a detailed fact sheet for community leaders, clinical protocols on partner violence and child abuse for health care professionals, and a self-learning module worth one Continuing Medical Education (CME) credit for physicians (authorized through 11/2001). It is geared to health care providers who wish to address family violence and promote family peace within a clinical setting. The site is sponsored by the Department of Family and Community Medicine, Medical College of Wisconsin.

The detailed clinical protocols, including general and specific signs indicating abuse, examples of how to take a comprehensive history of abuse, and specific information on how to help an adult victim of partner violence, are not readily found through other Web sites. It is unfortunate that this site does not provide links to other sites, particularly for consumers. Information is available only in English. The site is intended for health care professionals and is written accordingly. It is easy to use, although it is not as professionally designed as other sites.

Family Violence Prevention Fund

http://www.fvpf.org

The FVPF site, sponsored by the Family Violence Prevention Fund, a nonprofit organization based in San Francisco, offers a comprehensive set of information for community organizers, members of the criminal justice system, health professionals, advocates, policymakers, and others working to end violence against women. Of particular interest to consumers are links to facts about violence, a pop quiz on family violence, stories about the struggles of real women, and links to other Web sites on family violence. The information is carefully referenced and current.

By organizing the information into different pages for a variety of target audiences, the FVPF site is able to provide the most relevant information for each group. For example, the fact sheet for health care professionals gives full citations to professional journals, whereas the fact sheet for laypeople is more general. Information concerning the rights of immigrant women is especially useful, given that the issue is rarely addressed by other organizations.

The Web site does not give information directly targeted to abused women. FVPF materials are available in Spanish; however, no portions of the Web site are written in Spanish. The information generally is targeted to professionals. The language used reflects this fact. This is an attractive, professional, and easy-to-navigate site.

Minnesota Center Against Violence and Abuse

http://www.mincava.umn.edu

A well-developed, award-winning site with extensive electronic resources for survivors and professionals that is user-friendly on the topic of violence and abuse. The Minnesota Center Against Violence and Abuse supports research, education, and access to violence-related resources. The site is produced by the social work department of the University of Minnesota. The Minnesota State Legislature funded the creation of the Minnesota Center Against Violence and Abuse. The intended audience is primarily the general public, including battered women. There are also resources for professionals, as well as links to professional organizations. This is an excellent, well-organized site, with current and accurate information.

The site has 15 resource articles for survivors; lists approximately 38 survivor Web sites, such as those sponsored by the American Bar Association (see separate entry) and the American Medical Association's safety tips to prevent rape and campus violence; and gives a tour of a battered women's shelter. Survivor resources include a safety plan, a warning of how an abuser can detect sites accessed, and instructions on how to clear a browser cache.

This reviewer found no weaknesses in the site except for one dead link to the discussion group.

Although the site is primarily in English, links are given to multilanguage resources online and in print, including Spanish, braille, Haitian Creole, and Vietnamese. This is one of the most comprehensive, easy-to-use resources for professionals, survivors, and their children, and if utilized it can make an impact on violence prevention. It loads quickly, has a simple, clean design, and provides 47 clickable links to important specific topics. It is capable of doing a search for specific information with the results of the search returning rapidly. This site received an award for excellence.

National Coalition Against Domestic Violence

http://ncadv.org

The National Coalition Against Domestic Violence (NCADV) is dedicated to the empowerment of battered women and their children. It is the only national organization of grassroots shelter and service programs for battered women and is supported by Soroptimist International. The NCADV site is intended for the general public, the media, battered women and their children, and member agencies and organizations. The site has many valuable resources for battered women and their children, such as access to cosmetic repair for removing scars of abuse, links to state domestic violence coalitions and local shelters, descriptions of the dynamics of domestic violence, ways to get help, an ongoing project for compiling the names of murder victims, and a roundup of legislative and public policies.

The most important feature on the site for survivors of abuse is access to cosmetic repair for removing scars of abuse, links to state domestic violence coalitions and local shelters, description of dynamics of DV, ways to get help, and ways to change one's Social Security number. Other important features are links providing voting records of state and national legislators on domestic violence legislation; lists of supportive legislators, actors, and musical artists; and the "Remember My Name" project, a registry of murder victims' names.

Information packets are available for order in six different languages, as well as braille and audiotape for the blind. There are simple, easy-to-use icons for obtaining information, and the language is easy to understand. The colors of light gold and purple are easy on the eyes, links are easy to follow, and information quality is accurate and helpful.

Women's Health/Violence Against Women: Medem.com

http://www.medem.com
(click on "Medical Library," then "Women's Health," then "Violence Against Women")

The Medem site ("Women's Health/Violence Against Women") pro-vides basic domestic violence information from a variety of leading professional medical organizations, including the American Medical Association, the American Academy of Pediatrics, and the American College of Obstetrics and Gynecology. Most of the pages at this site are intended for consumers. A rating guide identifies four levels of complexity for each page, from "basic information" to "professional/research." The Violence against Women pages are at the second ("general health information") and third ("advanced resources") levels. This information is reasonably accurate. The sites do not discuss safety planning and they fail to emphasize the danger a woman faces in deciding to leave. Several of the links are out of date. Because of the authority conveyed by these medical societies, it is important that they have chosen to include sites on violence against women. As mentioned, the pages all fail to discuss safety planning for abused women, which is an important gap in a site addressed largely to abused women. Additionally, most pages do not direct women to discuss abuse with their physician, or lead women to expect their physician to broach the subject. Information on this site is available only in English. These pages are generally written at a basic reading level appropriate for general consumer use. The sites are easy to navigate. The information on violence against women is found under "women's health" within the "medical library."

REFERENCES

Campbell, J. (1998). *Empowering survivors of abuse.* Thousand Oaks: Sage.

Duffy, S., McGrath, M. D., Becker, B. M., & Linakis, J. G. (1999). Mothers with histories of domestic violence in a pediatric emergency department. *Pediatrics, 103,* 1007–1013.

Gazmararian, J. A., Lazorick, S., Spitz, A. M., Ballard, T. J., Saltzman, L. E., & Marks, J. S. (1996). Prevalence of violence against pregnant women. *Journal of the American Medical Association, 275,* 1915–1920.

Hotch, D., Grunfeld, A. F., Mackay, K., & Cowan, L. (1996). An emergency department based domestic violence intervention program: Findings after one year. *The Journal of Emergency Medicine, 14,* 111–117.

Plichta, S. B. (1997). Violence, health and the use of health services. In M. Falik & K. Collins (Eds.), *Women's Health: The Commonwealth Fund Survey* (pp. 237–272). Baltimore, MD: Johns Hopkins University Press.

_____ Chapter **13**

Drug and Alcohol Abuse

Kristen S. Montgomery, PhD, RNC, IBCLC

T he following Web sites offer information for those struggling with drug or alcohol abuse and access to the resources they need as they move toward recovery.

Alcoholics Anonymous

http://alcoholics-anonymous.org

Alcoholics Anonymous (AA) provides information and support regarding alcohol abuse. The site is intended for consumers and offers current and accurate information. Highlights include a fact file, information to help individuals determine if AA is right for them, a teen section, information for new members and individuals making referrals to AA (e.g., family members), contact information, and past meetings in a print newsletter format. The only weak point is that no additional information is provided about local AA activities; these are discussed in separate local Web pages. Information is provided in English, Spanish, and French. The reading level is simple to average. The site is easy to navigate, and information is presented in a nonjudgmental way.

Cocaine Anonymous World Services Online

http://www.ca.org

Cocaine Anonymous World Services Online is a support and networking site for individuals who have experienced cocaine addiction and wish to remain drug-free. The site is not affiliated with any sect, denomination, political party, or organization, but is supported through the contributions of members. No contribution is required, however, to be a member. Cocaine Anonymous supports a 12-step recovery program. The site is intended for consumers. Minimal content on drug abuse is found within the text, but what is presented is accurate and current. The focus of the site is geared to support of individuals as they recover from cocaine addiction.

The best features of the site include local telephone numbers and Web links, a self-test for cocaine addiction, a public information fact file, an outline of the 12 steps of the program, a section for newcomers, a section on crack news, and a meeting starter kit. The site ensures the confidentiality of individuals who access it. There are no weak points, although users should be aware that the 12-step program does include a religious component. The site is available in English and French. Content is at an average reading level, and the site is easy to use.

Drug Addiction Rehabilitation Institute

http://www.innovativetreatment.org

This Web site is an important resource for individuals searching for addiction treatment information. The purpose of the site is to provide information on top substance abuse treatment centers that meet a standard of high-quality treatment. Information is provided on treatment methods, cost, and rates of success. An extensive database is in progress; the site currently includes information on and links to Mountainside, Hazelden, Betty Ford, Narconon, LaHacienda, and Progressive Valley II–Women's Residence treatment centers. Consumers are the intended audience. Information is accurate and current. The only weakness of the site is the lack of information on drug addiction—only treatment options are provided. Information is available in English and is written at an average reading level. The site is easy to use.

Fetal Alcohol Syndrome Assistance and Training

http://home.golden.net/~fasat

Fetal Alcohol Syndrome Assistance and Training (FASAT) is a nonprofit organization dedicated to developing efficient and effective community responses for children with fetal alcohol syndrome/effects (FAS/E). The purpose of the site is to provide information, support, and resources for parents. The site is sponsored by FASAT, a partnership between professionals and parents in southern Ontario. The intended audience is consumers, specifically, parents. The information is useful and accurate. The best features of the site are a search mechanism, signs and symptoms of FAS/E (including pictures), common misconceptions, common questions and answers, training session information and fees, and information on parent support groups. The one weakness of the site is that only local information is included for support groups. The text is available only in English and is written at a simple to average level. The site is easy to use.

Narconon—Reducing the Drug Problem

http://www.narconon.org

Narconon is an information site on the Narconon way to stop using drugs, which focuses on communication, clean and ethical life, helping others, and family, friends, and society. Consumers are the intended audience, and Narconon sponsors the site. Information provided on the site is current and accurate. The best features of the site include drug facts, living without drugs, drug education, and celebrities' stories. There is also a "What's New" section for frequent users. There are no weaknesses to this site. Information is provided in English and at an average language level. The site is easy to navigate.

National Institute of Drug Addiction: Principles of Drug Addiction Treatment

http://www.nida.nih.gov/PODAT/PODATindex.html

The National Institute of Drug Addiction: Principles of Drug Addiction Treatment Web site is an information resource for the treatment of drug addiction. Information is provided in a question-and-answer format. The National Institute of Drug Addiction produces the site. It is unclear exactly to whom the content is geared; however, content is appropriate for consumers. Information is accurate and current. The best feature

Chapter 14

Elders and Their Families

Linda J. O'Connor, MSN, RNC, CS

This chapter lists sites specifically for elders, their families, and caregivers. The sites selected offer information on a wide range of topics in gerontology and elder care. They also provide a plethora of knowledge for health care professionals. For additional sites relevant to elders, see Chapter 37.

Age Concern

http://www.ace.org.uk

This international Web site is the home of Age Concern, which has 100 chapters throughout the United Kingdom and provides information on a multitude of issues concerning elders and their families. The site is for elders, their families, and caregivers, but it is also useful for health care professionals.

The "Facts for You" section comprises fact sheets on topics for elders and their families, reading lists, relevant Web links, and books for people over 50 and those who work with them.

This site provides excellent, easy-to-read information in a well-organized manner.

American Association for Retired Persons

http://www.aarp.org

See review in Chapter 37.

Caregivers.com

http://www.caregivers.com

This site is sponsored by AgeNet and provides information that can assist seniors and their families with the normal aging process. The text is in an easy-to-read, large-print format. The layout is organized and easy to navigate.

One of the highlights of this site is the section "Geriatrician Search," which provides a listing of geriatricians by state. Names, credentials, addresses, fax and phone numbers, and e-mail addresses are given. This section also provides a registration site for geriatricians who would like to be added to the listing.

Elderpage: Information for Older Persons and Families

http://www.aoa.dhhs.gov/elderpage.html

See review in Chapter 37.

Elderweb

http://www.elderweb.com

See review in Chapter 37.

Empowering Caregivers

http://www.care-givers.com

This is for caregivers providing care to people of all ages. The text is in large print, and the site is easily read and well indexed for navigation. The "Elder Links" section is an excellent page for caregivers of elders to bookmark. This section, which covers elder care, has an extensive listing and direct links to the major elder sites on the Internet. The site's sponsor is Gail Mitchell, who developed the site after she experienced personal loss following caregiving.

National Association on HIV Over Fifty

http://www.hivoverfifty.org

The mission of the National Association on HIV Over Fifty is to "promote the availability of a full range of educational, prevention, service, and health care programs for persons over age 50 affected by HIV." The organization's Web site is a starting place for elders affected by HIV, their health care providers, and caregivers. The site offers excellent fact sheets, an extensive bibliography, resource listings, and contacts across the United States, as well as links to other Web sites that provide HIV/AIDS information for elders.

The text is in large print, and the site is well organized.

Senior Cyborgs

http://www.online96.com/seniors

Senior Cyborgs is for people age 50 and over, their caregivers, and people who care for elders. The site covers a plethora of information that is of importance to seniors. It is organized into 25 different sections, including health and medicine, politics and government, fun and leisure, pets, a senior chat room, housing and retirement, death and dying, interesting links, and gerontology. This is an excellent site for elders that views aging as a normal, natural, healthy process. It is maintained by On-line Information Technology. Information on the site is managed by Elizabeth Alessio, MA, CSW, LNHA, a social worker.

Chapter 15

End-of-Life Care

Marianne LaPorte Matzo, PhD, RN, CS, GNP

The Internet is a new knowledge base on death and dying for health professionals, caregivers, family members, and the terminally ill. The following Web sites all offer useful information.

Choice in Dying

http://www.choices.org

Choice in Dying is dedicated to fostering communication about complex end-of-life decisions. The nonprofit organization provides advance directives, counsels patients and families, trains professionals, advocates for improved laws, and offers a range of publications and services. Choice in Dying devotes itself to ensuring that dying people are treated with dignity and respect, advocating for individuals' rights to participate fully in decisions about their medical treatment at the end of life, and securing the rights of people who need to receive adequate pain medication and other appropriate palliative treatment. The site offers a historical perspective on the right to die movement and differentiates between assisted suicide and euthanasia. The information is accurate and up to date. The legal section lets consumers look up information related to advance directives in their own state and to download those documents.

Death and Dying

http://death.net

Being terminally ill may make you feel like a stranger to the rest of society. You have to live differently, and most likely you will look at life differently. This site provides information and support to help individuals and their families through the trials of being terminally ill. The Web site includes chat areas, message boards in English and Spanish, and funeral planning guides. There are areas for children and even an area for relaxation called "The Fun Zone" that includes "The Escape Place," which offers games, polls, and surveys for your enjoyment. The site is owned and operated by Kelasan, Inc. It is designed to help the patient get through the hard times, meet others going through the same experiences, and find information and answers to questions. It is a very user-friendly site with current and pertinent information for terminally ill people and their families.

Funeral.com

http://www.funeral.com

Funeral.com reviews 125 decisions required when planning a funeral. The multitude of services and products involved in this process are organized into a simple 10-step process. Upon choosing the services they prefer, users can share their choices with other family members, save their choices at *funeral.com* for future consideration, or send their plan to the funeral home of their choice. There are many links and resources related to the social and cultural aspects of death and dying.

GriefNet

http://www.griefnet.org

GriefNet is an Internet community of persons dealing with grief, death, and major loss. There are 37 *support/index.html* e-mail support groups and two Web sites. The integrated approach to online grief support helps users work through their loss and grief issues. The companion site, *http://kidsaid.com*, provides a safe environment for kids and their parents to find information and ask questions. Cendra Lynn, PhD, a clinical grief psychologist, death educator, and traumatologist, super-vises GriefNet. GriefNet is supported by the donations of individuals and organizations and is operated as a nonprofit corporation under the name Rivendell Resources.

The Hemlock Society

http://www.hemlock.org

Founded in 1980 by Derek Humphry, the Hemlock Society is the oldest and largest right-to-die organization in the United States, and with more than 27,000 members in chapters across the country. The Hemlock Society shares information accumulated over almost 20 years on the options for a peaceful death. There are two parts to the organization: The Hemlock Foundation oversees publications, community services, such as the Patient Advocacy and Caring Friends programs, and re-search and charitable services. The Hemlock Society USA is the mem-bership arm and funds efforts to change the law related to assisted suicide. The Hemlock Society believes that people who wish to retain their dignity and choice at the end of life should have the option of a peaceful, gentle, certain, and swift death in the company of their loved ones. They believe the means to accomplish this is with legally pre-scribed medication as part of the continuum of care between a patient and a doctor.

Whether you are looking for background and current interests in the right to die movement, written information on planning for a peaceful death, or general information about the Hemlock Society, you should be able to find it at this Web site. The Hemlock Society's interest is in maximizing the options for a peaceful death, including legal physician aid in dying for terminally ill, mentally competent adults who request it, under careful safeguards. The Hemlock Society discourages suicide for emotional reasons; it does not dispense poisons or pills. The site offers trained Caring Friends volunteers and a professional Caring Friends team, who are ready to work with Hemlock members with terminal illnesses who are considering a hastened death and want the counseling and companionship offered by this program. The purpose of Caring Friends is to ensure that Hemlock members do not die alone, do not make failed attempts at self-deliverance, and have explored all alternatives. There is also a Hemlock Patient Advocacy Program to help ensure that living wills are followed. Although this site offers pertinent information, it is supportive of assisted suicide; persons unfamiliar with this topic can learn about the associated issues at this site.

Hospice Net—Death and Dying, Caregiving, and Grief

http://www.hospicenet.org

Hospice Net provides information and support to patients and families facing life-threatening illnesses. It is an independent, nonprofit 501(c)(3) organization working exclusively through the Internet. The site is divided into four parts: Services, Patients, Caregivers, and Bereavement. The Service section answers questions about the hospice concept and the services that are offered. The Patients Section offers information about advance directives and pain relief and includes the "Dying Person's Guide to Dying." Information for caregivers addresses how to help someone who is dying, how to say good-bye, and how to help a coworker. The section on bereavement has a guide to grief that will help individuals understand the grief that they may feel after a death, whether sudden or anticipated. There are areas for talking with children about death, children and grief, and helping teenagers cope with grief. The information is well organized, current, and accurate. The site is easily navigated, with appropriate links available.

Lastacts: A National Coalition to Improve Care and Caregiving at the End of Life

http://www.lastacts.org

See review in Chapter 37, "Long-Term-Care Services."

Links 2 Go: Death and Dying

http://www.links2go.com/topic/Death_and_Dying

Links2Go, with patent-protected technology, automatically compiles and prioritizes links to the most relevant Internet content on tens of thousands of topics spanning tens of millions of Web pages. The visitor can chat in real time about death and dying and related topics, view discussions related to this topic, and post new messages to the discussion. The links take the consumer through what appears to be every conceivable link related to death and dying. Resources found at this Web site were not available on other sites.

Pain Medicine and Palliative Care

http://www.wehealny.org/services/pain/index.html

This site is a part of the Continuum Health Partners Inc. health information Web site. Continuum Health Partners was formed in January 1997 as a partnership between two health care providers, Beth Israel Medical Center and St. Luke's–Roosevelt Hospital Center, both in New York. In May 1998 the partnership was joined by the Long Island College Hospital and more recently by the New York Eye and Ear Infirmary. The site has answers to frequently asked questions about end-of-life care, hospice, pain management, and palliative care. The information is accurate, and specific programs in the greater metropolitan New York area are highlighted.

Partnership for Caring: America's Voices for the Dying

http://www.partnershipforcaring.org

Partnership for Caring: America's Voices for the Dying is a national, nonprofit organization devoted to raising consumer expectations and increasing the demand for excellent care at the end of life. It is a consumer movement dedicated to increasing Americans' awareness of the challenges and opportunities associated with life's end and to removing the obstacles and building the skills required to meet those challenges and realize those opportunities. Information on this site refers to current legislation affecting the care provided at the end of life and provides the mechanism for involvement in these issues. An important feature of this site is the dissemination of the evolving end-of-life legislative agenda, with concrete ways for consumers to be involved.

Social Issues and Social Services: Death and Dying

http://www.mel.lib.mi.us/social/SOC-death.html

Michigan Electronic Library has listed links on topics related to the funeral home industry, euthanasia and assisted suicide, "death with dignity," and bereavement. This makes navigation quick and easy and allows users to link to a large number of resources.

Chapter 16

Environmental Health

Kathleen M. McPhaul, MPH, RN

E nvironmental health is an often-overlooked aspect of human health. Increasingly, communities and citizens are concerned about the environment; therefore, environmental health must concern health professionals as well. Most health professionals have not received adequate preparation or training in the principles of environmental health, but that will not stop consumers and patients from seeking information. The intent of the following reviews is to give a quick guide to some of the most valuable information on environmental health available on the Internet.

Consumers need environmental health information about their homes, schools, workplaces, and communities. They may be wondering about the safety of their food, drinking water, air, and even the soil near their homes. Furthermore, pregnant women, children, the elderly, the immunosuppressed, and the chronically ill are more vulnerable to environmental hazards. Finally, certain medical conditions, such as asthma and allergies, developmental and neurological conditions, and cancer, may be exacerbated or even caused by environmental contaminants. When questions arise about the health hazards associated with the environment, consider these Web sites as sources of accurate, timely, and credible information for consumers. The list does not do justice to the many other informative and credible sites; however, all of these sites link to even more specialized information, so don't be afraid to surf for yourself.

Agency for Toxic Substances and Disease Registry (ATSDR): ToxFAQs

http://www.atsdr.cdc.gov/toxfaq.html

ATSDR ToxFAQs is a series of summaries on hazardous substances and includes toxicological profiles, frequently asked questions about exposure, information on hazardous waste sites, human health effects, and public health statements. Its purpose is to provide substance-specific, easily understood information on chemicals known to be associated with hazardous waste sites. Its intended audience is consumers.

The Agency for Toxic Substances and Disease Registry was created to assess human health issues associated with hazardous waste sites. It is an agency within the federal Centers for Disease Control.

The information is accurate, but new information is added slowly. The agency has created easy-to-understand fact sheets (ToxFAQs) on many important and hazardous chemicals. They are listed alphabetically.

The ToxFAQ page is well organized for its purpose. If the consumer expects to get locality-specific chemical-release information, however, the main ATSDR Web site is too difficult to navigate and too poorly organized. The EPA Envirofacts page (*http://www.epa.gov/epahome/comm.htm*) and the Environmental Defense Fund's Scorecard (*http://www.scorecard.org*) are better options for consumers who want locality-specific information.

Consumers also can link to the ATSDR/EPA's "Top 20 Hazardous Substances List D" (*http://www.atsdr.cdc.gov/toxfaq.html*) and the "Medical Management Guidelines for Acute Chemical Exposures: Patient Information" (*http://www.atsdr.cdc.gov/mmg.html*), provided in this file, in a straightforward and user-friendly, question/answer format.

The Association of Occupational and Environmental Clinics

http://www.aoec.org

The Association of Occupational and Environmental Clinics (AOEC) is a network of more than 60 clinics and 250 individuals committed to improving the practice of occupational and environmental medicine through information sharing and collaborative research. The long-term goal of AOEC is to facilitate the prevention and treatment of occupational and environmental illnesses and injuries through collaborative reporting and investigation of health problems.

The purpose of the site is to enhance communication among member clinics and general membership. There is a complete list of the member clinics and contact information. The site is produced by the AOEC, with additional federal funding from the Agency for Toxic Substances and Disease Registry and the National Institutes of Occupational Safety and Health. The intended audience is AOEC membership. The clinic directory is useful to consumers because consumers often have difficulty finding providers familiar with environmental disease and their assessment. The AOEC also has established a network of Pediatric Environmental Specialty units throughout the nation. The clinic contact information is accurate and timely.

The site reflects the high standards of the organization. It provides a complete list of occupational/environmental and pediatric/environmental specialty units. It is a very trustworthy source of referral clinics.

However, the site is awkward to navigate and organized for its chief purpose, communication among members. Locating the clinic directory requires reading the descriptive text. There are no navigational buttons for quick access to sections. Clinic contact information does not include links to clinic Web pages. Information is in English only.

Although this is not the most visually appealing or sophisticated of Web sites, it does provide a complete clinic directory of its members. The AOEC is an environmental/occupational clinic organization requiring competency and ethical standards from its member clinics. The clinics are consumer/patient-centered. Unfortunately, with fewer than 75 clinics, not all consumers will be close to a site. Phone consultations are usually possible between health care providers.

The Children's Environmental Health Network

http://www.cehn.org

The Children's Environmental Health Network (CEHN) is a national multidisciplinary project whose mission is to promote a healthy environment and protect the fetus and the child from environmental health hazards. This site provides information on the Children's Environmental Health Network, the organizations' publications and activities, and links to sources of information and resources in the field. The intended audience is consumers, parents, children's health advocates, and health providers.

"Tips for Parents and Caregivers" (*cehn/Tips.html*) is a link showing a list of things that consumers can do to better protect children. The "Resource Guide on Children's Environmental Health" (*cehn/resourceguide/rghome.html*) is an impressive compilation of profiles of resource organizations and projects. You can search by organization or by toxicant. The site has no substantial weaknesses; however, as the premier advocacy organization for children's environmental health, the CEHN site should provide more bilingual information. As is, information is in English only.

Environmental Protection Agency: Concerned Citizens Resources

http://www.epa.gov/epapages/epahome/citizen.htm

This is a consumer-oriented gateway to the U.S. Environmental Protection Agency's massive Web site and other Web-based and print resources on environmental health. The site helps users become familiar with environmental issues and potential environmental and human health risks caused by pollution.

Section links include "Community Right-to-Know," "Protecting Our Children," "At Home and in the Garden," "At the Workplace," "Transportation," "Resources to Nonprofit Organizations," "Thinking Globally, Acting Locally," "Environmental Violations," and "Environmental Emergencies."

This site is the federal government's official source of information on the environment and is highly accurate and timely. Pages include the date of last update.

The best features include direct links to other parts of EPA Web sites especially the colorful Office of Children's Health Protection Web page (*http://www.epa.gov/children*), the consumer oriented section on pesticides and food (*http://www.epa.gov/pesticides/food*), the zip code–specific air and watershed data section, Envirofacts (*http://www.epa.gov/epahome/comm.htm*), and the drinking water sites that link to each state's public drinking water information office (*http://www.epa.gov/safewater/dwinfo.htm* and *http://www.epa.gov/safewater/dwhealth.html*).

The novice user may be overwhelmed by the vast amount of information here. The Citizen's Resources page is well organized. However, it is easy to tunnel very deep into the Web site and became disoriented. The viewer can always return to the EPA homepage but may need to repaste the address or bookmark the Concerned Citizen's Resource gateway. The site is in English only. A few publications are offered in Spanish.

The information is exceptional in content, the visual layout of most pages is appealing and well organized, and the complexity of the information ranges from very simple to very technical and complex. Most users will be able to understand the sections devoted to consumers. The EPA Web site will alert consumers to links outside the site.

Farm-A-Syst Home-A-Syst: Help Yourself to a Healthy Home

http://www.uwex.edu/homeasyst

This site educates homeowners and consumers about home environmental hazards, including how to assess hazards and develop a plan to reduce environmental hazards. It presents simple and practical solutions for consumers.

Home-A-Syst is a national program supported by the U.S. Department of Agriculture (USDA) Cooperative State Research, Education, and Extension Service (CSREES), the USDA Natural Resources Conservation Service (NRCS), and the U.S. Environmental Protection Agency (EPA).

The information is highly accurate and timely. This site is focused on the consumer, so the text is simple and practical. It is one of the few sites that takes a comprehensive view of the home and includes both assessment and practical solutions. Information is given in a clear, concise, and colorful way.

The best features include the brochures that are fully downloaded from the Web:

- *Help Yourself to a Healthy Home: Protect Your Children's Health* discusses indoor air quality, hazardous household products, and problems with lead, pesticides, and drinking water. The booklet is also available in Spanish.
- *Home-A-Syst: An Environmental Risk-Assessment Guide for the Home* provides links to many more resources on environmental hazards in the home and Home-A-Syst program contacts in each state.

It is difficult to understand the structure and mission of the Home-A-Syst program. The sponsoring agencies and funding sources are clear, but the purpose, mission, and structure of the organization are not explicit. Most of this information is in the "Threshold" newsletter and "Info for Educators" section. The labeling of the buttons on the homepage is vague.

This site and its publications cover all the environmental hazards in the home. These resources are specifically designed for consumers. There are government resources for home environmental health, but they are topic specific, such as the Housing and Urban Development's Web site for lead in homes (*http://www.hud.gov/hhchild.html*) and the EPA's site on indoor air quality (*http://www.epa.gov/iaq/homes.html*).

OSHA's Worker Page

http://www.osha.gov/as/opa/worker/index.html

This is the worker section of the Web site of the Occupational Safety and Health Agency (OSHA). The OSHA Worker Page houses information on workers' rights under the Occupational Safety and Health Act and provides information and guidance on how to exercise those rights. It is sponsored by the U.S. Department of Labor, Occupational Safety and Health Agency. The intended audience is workers.

Information is timely and accurate. The best feature is the question-and-answer format on workers' rights and responsibilities.

The site could be improved by including or linking to the well-developed training and outreach activities of the agency. Another deficiency is there is no explanation or link to the OSHA inspection database so that workers can view their employers' or their particular industry's inspection history. Finally, the site does not provide information on high-risk jobs or high-risk industry sectors. The workers' page should include a summary of the injury data collected by the agency.

OSHA has a well-developed training and outreach mandate and substantial information on its training Web page (*http://www.osha-slc.gov/Training*). These training and outreach activities should also be linked to the worker page and an effort made to tailor these activities to workers, health and safety committees, and worker's advocacy groups, such as unions.

Chapter 17

Exercise and Physical Fitness

Kristine M. C. Talley, BSN, RN and
Jean F. Wyman, PhD, RN, CS, FAAN

A selection of exercise and physical fitness-related Web sites from nonprofit, governmental, and commercial organizations are reviewed in this section. The sites were chosen based on their potential interest to consumers and health educators, as well as on the accuracy and usefulness of their content. Health educators will find information useful for designing education material on general physical fitness and exercise and on exercising with special health conditions, such as diabetes and pregnancy. Consumers will find information on how to start and maintain an exercise program and how to select a fitness trainer. Beginning exercisers will find all the sites informative and motivating, whereas advanced exercisers will find the two commercial Web sites, *http://walking.about.com* and *http://thriveonline.oxygen. com/fitness*, more appealing. The commercial sites have chat rooms and forums that consumers can use to troubleshoot exercise barriers and to create an environment supportive of exercise. Most of the sites also provide links to other Web sites, thus expanding their scope of information. Although this is not an exhaustive list of exercise sites, it does provide reputable and accurate information on exercise and physical fitness and is useful for beginning, intermediate, and advanced exercisers, as well as for health educators.

About.com: Walking Section

http://walking.about.com

About: The Human Internet is a publicly held Internet company that builds comprehensive Web sites on specific topics. Walking is one of the organization's 700 guide sites. This site has much to offer walkers of all levels. There are tips to help beginners, as well as information for people who want to advance to racewalking or marathon walking. The Web site provides links to related sites and high-quality original content on walking. Walkers can use this site to find walking clubs, log on to scheduled chat sessions, and post walking-related questions on forum bulletin boards. There are links to catalogs to purchase recommended walking equipment (i.e., clothing and shoes) and books about walking. The linked sites are reputable; for example, there is a link to the American Orthopedic Foot and Ankle Society site, which demonstrates proper stretching. The site is moderately easy to use. There is an alphabetized subject list on the left side of the screen. However, there are times when linked sites do not allow users to click on the "back" button to return to the *walking.about.com* Web site. There is also a great deal of information and graphics on the site, so it can take time to download pages.

This is a valuable site for anyone who walks or wants to begin a walking program. It serves as a resource to solve problems in a walking program and to help keep walkers motivated to continue and progress with their exercise.

American Council on Exercise

http://www.acefitness.org

The site is produced by the American Council on Exercise (ACE), a nonprofit organization that sets certification and education standards for fitness instructors. There is information valuable to both fitness experts and consumers. Consumers can use this site to find certified fitness trainers and facilities. The most useful feature for consumers is the "ACE Fit Facts," which covers over 80 fact sheets on a multitude of fitness issues. It is one of the few sites that provide tips on how to exercise safely with health challenges, such as diabetes, asthma, and arthritis. The "ACE Fit Tips" are useful to learn about new exercise activities and to help overcome barriers to exercise. The level of information is simple to average. The site is easy to use. There is a menu list of different topics included on the left side of the screen. There are no interactive tools for consumers. The site also sells fitness books, most of which appeal to fitness trainers. Consumers can sign up to receive a free monthly *ACE Health E-tips* newsletter. Most of the site is dedicated to helping fitness trainers and facilities to become certified.

However, consumers may find some of the certification information useful for evaluating the quality of their own exercise trainers.

Exercise and Your Heart: A Guide to Physical Activity

http://www.nih.gov/health/exercise/index.htm

This site is an online version of a pamphlet developed jointly by the National Institutes of Health and the National Heart, Lung, and Blood Institute. It provides up-to-date information on the effects of physical activity on the heart as well as practical guidelines for starting and staying with an exercise program. The site accurately describes the impact of inactivity on health, particularly on the heart, stresses the benefits of regular physical activity, and provides examples of how many calories are consumed with particular activities. It debunks common myths about exercise and helps create solutions to exercise barriers. A table explains target heart rate values. There are two sample activity programs that give detailed guidelines on how to start a walking or jogging program.

The format of the site is pure text. There are no pictures or interactive tools. However, the information included is accurate, and the site's producers are reputable. There is no advertising on the site or links to other exercise Web pages.

This site is most useful for individuals who are recovering from a heart attack and for beginning exercisers.

Fitness Overview: Medem.com

http://www.medem.com
(click on "Medical Library," then "Fitness and Nutrition," then "Fitness Overview")

Medem.com is a commercial Internet site founded by seven of the nation's top medical societies. Some of the founders include the American Medical Association, the American Psychiatric Association, and the American College of Obstetricians and Gynecologists. The Web site provides a medical library composed of health-related articles provided by and approved by these medical societies. There are two ways to access fitness information. The first, and easiest way, is to click on "Medical Library," then "Fitness and Nutrition," then "Fitness Overview."

This retrieves 10 articles on basic fitness, including an introduction to fitness, starting an exercise program, and sticking with it. The second way to access fitness information is to type the word "fitness" into the "search medical library" prompt on the home page. This retrieves a list of over 100 articles on various aspects of fitness. There is useful information about exercising with special medical conditions, such as diabetes, pregnancy, and arthritis. The peer-review system used by the site's founders ensures that information is accurate. Articles include safety precautions to follow when beginning or maintaining an exercise program. Using the site is relatively easy. Before the title of each article is a rating symbol, which indicates if the article contains introductory health information, general health information, advanced resources, or professional/research. Even with the indicator symbol it can be a bit time consuming to locate the article of interest. One advantage of the site is the absence of advertising material, which is unique for a commercial Web site. Health care professionals will find useful research articles, as well as general and specific fitness information that can be used for client education. The site is also recommended to consumers seeking basic or advanced information about fitness and exercise.

MEDLINEplus: Exercise/Physical Fitness Section

http://www.nlm.nih.gov/medlineplus/exercisephysicalfitness.html

MEDLINEplus (see general review in Chapter 1) created this Web page to provide health care professionals and consumers with links to sites on exercise and physical fitness. The list is categorized to help the reader select relevant sites. For example, there are categories specific to exercise recommendations for women, children, and seniors. There is also a list of sites that provide exercise recommendations for specific health conditions, such as osteoporosis and asthma. There is even a category for exercise Web sites created in Spanish. Most of the linked sites are part of the National Library of Medicine at the National Institutes of Health, so users can be assured of receiving high-quality information on exercise and fitness. The linked sites vary in the level of information provided. Some sites give comprehensive information on starting a fitness routine, whereas others provide information on specific components of fitness, such as what to eat before exercising. MEDLINEplus follows strict selection guidelines when deciding what information to include on the Web page; therefore, the linked sites give information that is up to date, accurate, and informative.

Advantages include the absence of advertising on the site and the fact that MEDLINEplus does not endorse any company or product. The site is updated frequently, and all the listed site addresses are accessible. A possible disadvantage is the lack of links to informative commercial sites. This is an excellent starting point for searching exercise and physical fitness Web sites.

Thriveonline: Fitness Section

http://thriveonline.oxygen.com/fitness

ThriveOnline was founded in 1996 as a joint venture between America Online and Time Inc. and is now a wholly owned subsidiary of Oxygen Media. The fitness section is one of six topics at *thriveonline.oxygen.com.* The fitness section's mission is to motivate people to participate in physical activity. Its target audience is active people looking for new types of workouts and beginners who need information, tips, and motivation to get started. There are pages dedicated to developing exercise routines for walking, running, cycling, toning, yoga, weight training, swimming, boxing, and pilates (pronounced pi-lah-tees—pilates is a series of body sculpting maneuvers that strengthens muscles, improves posture, and tones midsection muscles without using weights). Routines are designed for beginning, intermediate, and advanced exercisers. Each exercise topic includes a section on warming up and cooling down and has photographs depicting individual exercises. There are also recommendations on overcoming common barriers to exercise. There are tips on how to fit exercise in at work, at home, and during pregnancy. The site also has some moderately useful interactive tools to determine target heart rates, body mass index, and calorie counts. However, this reviewer did not find the "Fitness Planner," "Breathing IQ Test," and "Muscle Match Game" useful.

The site provides access to chat rooms and expert advice. Karen Voight, a nationally known fitness consultant and personal trainer, answers users' questions. There are also other experts such as nutritionists available to answer questions. Only the most common or interesting questions get a published answer, and the questions are not updated frequently.

There is some difficulty in maneuvering from page to page. Each topic page has a different format, and there is no easy way to get back to the fitness homepage without returning to the main page.

This site is very useful for helping beginners to design an exercise program and for motivating current exercisers to continue.

Chapter 18

Genetics

Felissa R. Lashley, PhD, RN, ACRN, FAAN

G enetics is becoming the key to understanding the causes of and possible therapies for many diseases, including breast cancer and Alzheimer's disease. With the map of the entire human genetic "blueprint" made possible by the Human Genome Project, this topic is of keen interest to health professionals and the general public. Many of the sites described here offer comprehensive information on genetics, in most cases more than the average consumer may want to know. However, interested individuals can find appropriate information on any related topic by seeking out the type of information needed and the level of presentation with which they are most comfortable.

Genetic Alliance

http://geneticalliance.org

This site emphasizes support groups and resources for consumers. It is sponsored by the Genetic Alliance (formerly the Alliance of Genetic Support Groups Inc.), an international coalition of individuals, professionals, and genetic support organizations that is working together to enhance the lives of everyone affected by genetic conditions. The site is for consumers, foundations, agencies, advocates, and health care professionals. Information appears current and accurate.

This site emphasizes support groups, resources, and public policy issues affecting individuals and families with genetic conditions. The

resources pages cover such diverse topics as bioethics, disability resources, ethnocultural issues, educational resources, grief and loss,
and professional societies.

The site is attractive and relatively easy to understand and use. It
gives links to sources in other languages, such as IDEXMEDICO, a
bilingual medical information service.

Genetics Education Center

http://www.kumc.edu/gec

This is a very comprehensive site emphasizing genetic education,
the Human Genome Project, and resources. It is sponsored by the
University of Kansas Medical Center.

The intended audience is educators interested in human genetics.
The site has comprehensive information not only about genetic education but also about genetic conditions and support groups and ways
to locate genetic experts. The information presented is current and accurate.

Resources pages cover genetic education information and material,
including curricula, lesson plans, hands-on materials, computer programs, and books and videotapes. The site also has information on
genetic conditions, careers, professional societies, and the Human
Genome Project. Information is in English only. The site is attractive
and easy to use.

Human Genome Project Information

http://www.ornl.gov/hgmis

This is an extremely comprehensive site, with both historical and current
information about the Human Genome Project and educational resources. It is produced by the U.S. Department of Energy. The site is
for professionals and consumers. Information is current and accurate.

In addition to the information on the Human Genome Project, including sequencing, mapping, and instrumentation, this site contains basic
information, such as "Genetics 101," a glossary, information on genetic
testing, gene therapy, pharmacogenomics, disease information, genetic counseling, ethical, legal, and social issues, forensic information,
genetics in the courtroom, and videos and other materials for teachers.

It has many useful links, including those to support groups. Information is in English only. The site is easy to use and can be searched using alphabetical and subject indices.

National Human Genome Research Institute

http://www.nhgri.nih.gov

This site provides comprehensive information on the Human Genome Project, as well as related research initiatives and genetic-related policies. It is produced by the National Human Genome Research Institute, part of the National Institutes of Health. The site is for researchers, professionals, and consumers. Information is current and accurate.

This is a major resource for understanding the goals and result of the Human Genome Project, including the ethical, legal, and social implications. The site emphasizes research and grant information, as well as policy issues and public affairs. It features a glossary and "In the News" section.

Office of Rare Diseases, National Institutes of Health

http://rarediseases.info.nih.gov/ord/

This site, produced by the National Institutes of Health, provides information on thousands of rare diseases (defined as affecting no more than 200,000 persons), many of which are genetic. The intended audience is professionals and consumers.

The site gives information on rare disease research studies and progress and includes a clinical research database. There is also a listing of genetic counselors and counseling centers, as well as information on travel and lodging for treatment and research sites. Links cover other genetic research information, health organizations, and terms and definitions, as well as the National Library of Medicine's PubMed. This is a relatively straightforward site that is easy to use.

Online Mendelian Inheritance in Man: National Center for Biotechnology Information

http://www.ncbi.nlm.nih.gov/omim

The major feature of this database is a comprehensive catalog of human genes and genetic disorders. The site is sponsored by the

National Center for Biotechnology Information. It is authored and edited by Victor A. McKusick and colleagues at Johns Hopkins University. The target audience is health professionals concerned with genetic disorders, genetic researchers, and advanced students. It is useful to consumers because of the accurate and comprehensive scientific and clinical information provided on virtually every known genetic condition.

The site's most important feature is the up-to-date information on thousands of genetic conditions and diseases that is searchable by condition or keyword. There are gene maps and important links and mutation databases on humans and animals. Information is in English only. The site is easy to use.

Chapter **19**

Heart Disease

Hussein A. Tahan, MS, RN, CNA

The Internet is changing how heart patients receive their care and health information. It is not unusual today for a patient or a family member to give a nurse or a physician documents related to heart disease printed off the Internet. Because health care consumers may not be as educated about or as aware of how to evaluate the resources available on the Internet, it is important for health professionals to assume some responsibility in this regard and to streamline the Internet information patients may encounter. It is imperative to do so because the quality of this information is critically important as it could affect the health care outcomes of millions of patients.

About 58 million Americans, almost one fourth of the nation's population, live with some form of heart disease. Among both men and women, and across all racial and ethnic groups, cardiovascular diseases (referring to a variety of diseases and conditions of the heart and vessels) is the nation's leading killer. It is estimated that 960,000 Americans die of cardiovascular disease each year. Eliminating cardiovascular disease would increase life expectancy by almost 10 years (CDC, 2000). The economic burden of this disease continues to grow as the population ages. Therefore, it is essential for health professionals and their patients to engage themselves in cardiovascular disease prevention and health promotion activities and to promote awareness of the risk factors for heart disease and the strategies to reduce such risk. There are 233,000 Web pages currently available specializing in heart disease, identified via the Yahoo search engine using the keyword "heart disease."

This chapter describes 10 Web sites covering cardiovascular-related consumer resources. They were selected for their reliable, credible, and current information. The online resources are extensive. Access to these sites is free of charge. Not all of the sites require special browser or explorer technology. Most honor the Health on the Net Foundation Code, and only one allows advertisements to a limited degree. In addition, they all include a disclaimer that advises site visitors to consult with a physician or a health care professional before implementing any of the recommendations on the site. Moreover, these Web sites use health care experts and professionals to develop the information they publish online or to act in an advisory or consultative role. The sites reviewed here present unique characteristics and nontraditional strategies for health promotion, maintenance, and disease prevention. Features include the following (not available on every Web site reviewed):

Chat rooms

Online synchronous and asynchronous support groups for counseling and emotional support

Animated and nonanimated educational materials

E-mail access to health care professionals for questions and answers

Dictionary of medical terms

Quizzes and tools for evaluating one's knowledge about heart disease

Real-life stories and experiences shared by real people suffering from heart disease

Availability of search engines

Online newsletters

American Heart Association

http://www.americanheart.org
http://www.americanheart.org/Heart_and_Stroke_A_Z_Guide

The American Heart Association (AHA) is a nonprofit professional association of physicians, nurses, and allied health professionals. Its mission is to fight heart disease and stroke. The AHA's Web site is oriented primarily toward health care professionals; however, it also includes some consumer-related features. These are:

- Warning Signs—discusses the signs and symptoms of heart attack and when to contact a physician
- Heart and Stroke A to Z Guide—presents patient, family, and caregiver instruction materials that are accessible through an alphabetical index of different topics
- Risk Awareness—explains the risk factors for heart disease, such as smoking, hypertension, weight, and high cholesterol. It also presents strategies to reduce these risks
- Family Health—discusses health promotion and disease prevention. Programs shared here include exercise, healthy cooking, smoking cessation, lifestyle management, and stress reduction
- Links—hyperlinks this site to related Web sites

Health care professionals may use the information shared on this Web site to educate patients, families, and caregivers regarding heart disease and its related diagnostic and therapeutic procedures and interventions. The "A to Z Guide" includes more than a thousand topics that are accessible via an alphabetical index. An important feature of this site is the inclusion of quizzes users can take to assess their own risk for heart disease. Although this information is credible, it is not clear when postings on the site were last updated. "Heart to Heart" electronic greeting cards are also available free of charge—users can send cards electronically to friends, families, and other patients.

Another important feature is the children-specific section, where topics specific to children, such as congenital heart diseases, are addressed. Information in this area is presented in a child-friendly way and includes illustrations; however, the language used may be too difficult for children to understand, which makes it essential for an adult to assist a child in navigating the site and explaining the information.

The AHA Web site is well organized; however, it includes extensive information that makes it difficult for less computer-literate consumers to navigate successfully. Although it includes consumer and professional features, this is not made evident on the main page. The search engine capability enhances the search function by topic. Navigating the site requires Netscape Navigator 3.0 or a later version or Internet Explorer 3.0 or later browser technology. Other browsers may not display the information properly, especially the information formatted in a table.

American Heart Association: Take Wellness to Heart Campaign

http://www.women.americanheart.org

The Take Wellness to Heart campaign is the American Heart Association's (AHA) site devoted exclusively to women's heart health. The site is developed by the AHA and is sponsored by Aetna US Healthcare and an unrestricted educational grant from Wyeth-Ayerst Laboratories. The mission of the campaign is to help women with or at risk for heart disease learn how to take care of themselves and their families and empower them to share heart health information with other women. Participation in this site requires users to fill out a registration form that consists of a demographic and contact information sheet and an assessment form that examines women's perception and knowledge of warning signs for and risk factors of heart disease. Registration allows users to receive announcements and information regarding the latest updates, links, and stories added to the site via e-mail.

The site includes the following sections:

- Know Heart and Stroke—includes information about cardiovascular disease, news releases, and recent related articles
- Take Wellness to Heart—shares information about the latest legislation and public advocacy, with sample letters to congressional representatives, and includes a women's event calendar, with information on heart walks and other community programs
- A Lighter Heart—includes tips for eating and cooking heart-healthy food, smoking cessation, and exercise. It also includes the "Women's Online Forum," through which women can share their stories and provide emotional support to each other. Another aspect of this feature is the "Heart to Heart" electronic cards that can be used as greeting messages
- Gatekeeper—provides educational materials and tips for staying healthy and reducing the risk for heart disease. It also provides information on pediatric heart disease, disease prevention, caregiver–related tips, and treating the elderly with heart disease
- Self-Care—features an extensive guide to risks for heart disease and the relationship between alcohol, oral contraceptives, menopause, and pregnancy and heart disease

A direct link to the AHA's Web site (see separate entry) is available on this site, where other related information is easily accessible. Although there is no search feature on the homepage, a search engine is available through the "Self-Care" section; however, it is limited to a preselected list of topics. This search capability resembles a list of hyperlinks to other areas of the Web site. An interesting aspect of this site is the use of tools such as a quiz and a screening form, where users can learn more about heart disease. Resources shared on this site are credible, clear, and simple. However, it is difficult to determine the currency of the information because no dates are available indicating when these resources were posted or last updated.

Children's Health Information Network

http://www.tchin.org

The Children's Health Information Network (CHIN) is a nonprofit organization created by the mother of a child with complex heart defects. The aim of this Web site is to provide information and resources to families of children with congenital and acquired heart disease, adults with congenital heart defects, and the professionals who work with them. The site is supported by donations from individuals, corporations, foundations, and educational grants. The educational information and support resources available on this site are developed and managed by volunteers who are physicians, nurses, allied health professionals, and nonprofessional persons. A board that consists of physicians and nurses specializing in pediatric cardiology advises and assists CHIN in developing, revising, and editing the patient education materials published on the site and previewing related Web sites before they are linked through the CHIN site.

CHIN features the following:

- Community—provides online support to children and their families using chat rooms that are available free of charge. This feature includes a family room through which patients and families can pose questions to other patients and families or respond to questions posed by others; a memorial garden, which includes pictures and short stories in memory of children who have died of congenital heart disease; a portrait gallery of children suffering from heart disease; and a teen lounge specific to teens to share their stories with others, ask questions, and respond to others' questions.
- Resources—includes reviews of books about congenital heart disease, as well as fiction and nonfiction children's books. It also

features a list of support groups that are available in the United States, Canada, and other countries. In addition, patient education materials related to certain topics and advertisements of special events such as regional conferences are accessible through this feature

- Internet links—houses hundreds of different hyperlinks to related Web sites and Internet resources. The links are important for patients and their families and health care professionals. These links are organized into nine categories, including adults with congenital heart disease, grief and bereavement, defects and syndrome specific, health care insurance, humanitarian organizations, Internet guides, summer camps, transplant resources, informational resources, and organizations
- Contact information—includes information about the advisory board, volunteers, events, donations, and awards received by CHIN

The site is easy to navigate. A site map is available at the bottom of the homepage. The information shared is credible, clear, and simple to understand. The site is patient- and family-focused and provides lots of avenues for support, including the chat room, e-mail, and support group capabilities. CHIN honors the Health on the Net Foundation Code and is a member of the Maternal Child Health (MCH) Web Ring, which is an Internet megasite sponsored by the Institute for Child Health Policy and supported by the MCH Bureau of the Department of Health and Human Services. To navigate the site, users need one of the following browsers: Netscape Communicator 2.0, 3.0, or 3.01 with Java, or Microsoft Internet Explorer 3.1, 3.01, or 3.01b.

HeartFailure Online

http://www.heartfailure.org

This Web site is sponsored by the Sharp Foundation of Cardiovascular Research and Education and the San Diego Cardiac Center, San Diego, CA. It is bilingual (English and Spanish) and dedicated to patients with heart failure. The site includes a search engine for searching either the site itself or the Net by topic.

HeartFailure Online does not have any advertisements. It consists of seven sections that provide patients and their families with heart failure-related information and educational materials. These are:

- How the Heart Works—includes information regarding the physiology of the heart and vessels
- What's Heart Failure?—defines heart failure, in particular, the different types of heart failure, and explains the related risk factors
- Do I Have Heart Failure?—discusses the signs and symptoms of heart failure and the tests used to diagnose the presence of the disease
- Living with Heart Failure—includes instructions on healthy lifestyle, medications intake, visiting the doctor, and weight monitoring
- What's New—presents the latest pharmaceutical treatment of heart failure and the use of the portable left ventricular assist device
- Frequently Asked Questions—lists the most common questions as a suggested list for patients to use when they visit their physicians
- Links to related sites—includes hyperlinks to other heart failure–specific sites, other cardiac-related sites, and select publications

The patient and family educational materials available on this site are written at a lower reading level and include illustrations where appropriate. The information shared is clear and concise; however, it is difficult to determine its currency because no dates are available that indicate when the information was posted online or last updated. Medication management and weight-monitoring charts are available for patients to print for their own use as needed. Certain topics, such as diet, exercise, and smoking cessation, are hyperlinked to related materials available on the American Heart Association Web site (see separate entry).

Heart Information Network

http://www.heartinfo.com

HeartInfo is an independent educational Web site developed by a patient and a physician. It provides a range of information and services to heart patients and others who are interested in lowering their risk status for heart disease. The site is easy to navigate and includes various features, including the following:

- Tell a Friend—is an e-mail medium among heart patients and health care providers

- Q&A library and frequently asked questions—presents a compilation of 1,000 questions asked by patients and their related answers as provided by physicians
- Find a Specialist—a directory of health care providers, facilities, and services specializing in heart failure, hypertension, and lipid care
- Nutrition guide—a guide to eating healthy and making dietary and lifestyle changes to improve heart health
- Risks—provides information sheets about the tests used to identify the risks for heart disease and strategies that can be applied to reduce these risks
- Patient's stories—includes a compilation of stories submitted by real patients describing their experiences and successes with heart disease
- Glossary of medical terms—an interpretation of medical terms using simple language
- Resources—provides information and educational material covering a multitude of diagnoses, treatments, and diagnostic tests. Almost all items are in English; a few are in Spanish, such as "heart attack symptoms"
- News—shares snapshots of the latest advances in the identification, treatment, and prevention of heart disease as they appear in other professional and lay media

An editorial board manages this site. Members of the board represent different specializations, such as medicine, nursing, nutrition, physical therapy, and pharmacy. The board also includes members who are not health care professionals. HeartInfo features a site map and a site-specific search engine, as well as hyperlinks to related Web sites. In addition, it includes an evaluative review of each of the hyperlinked sites, applying a set of criteria developed by the HeartInfo staff. The resources available on this site are clear, simple, credible, and current. The site indicates the date of the last update made to the information. No advertisements are included except for special resources/programs available on the site, such as "Understanding Blood Pressure" and "Cardio Fit."

HeartPoint

http://www.heartpoint.com

The HeartPoint Web site provides patients and their families with credible information and educational material specific to heart disease. The site was developed by medical professionals, is owned and maintained by a physician specializing in heart disease, and is sponsored by Medtronic and Hoechst Marion Roussell Inc. This site honors the Health on the Net Foundation Code. The various features of the HeartPoint Web site are:

- HeartPoint Gallery—provides educational materials explaining various aspects of the heart and diagnostic and therapeutic modalities of caring for heart disease
- Health Tips—shares brief rundowns and checklists of important topics on health and health care, such as medication management and questions to ask during a doctor's visit
- Food You Will Love—provides recipes for heart-smart cooking and healthy eating
- In the News—covers important subjects about cardiac care and the latest treatment innovations
- What's New—alerts site visitors to what is new, as well as upcoming features
- Information Center—houses the site map, contact information, archives, and links to other sites

Patients, families, and caregivers can access educational information on more than 30 different heart disease topics by clicking on the "HeartPoint Gallery" icon. This information is credible, clear, simple, and current. The homepage includes the date of the last update made to the site. The use of animated graphics is a pleasant and amusing feature of this site's library of information. Each topic includes other related subtopics, and, where appropriate, strategies for health management and lifestyle changes are shared (e.g., a contract for weight loss programs and a quiz for smoking cessation that help identify the best strategies a patient may adopt). HeartPoint does not include a site map; however, it provides a search engine feature to locate information on a topic of interest. Users also can search current and archived information. HeartPoint requires Internet Explorer 3.0 or later for site navigation.

Johns Hopkins Heart Health: Patient Information

http://www.jhbmc.jhu.edu/cardiology/rehab/patientinfo.html

This Web site is developed by the Johns Hopkins Bayview Medical Center's Division of Cardiology, Cardiac Rehabilitation, and Prevention and sponsored by the medical center. It is accessible independently at the above URL address or through the medical center's Web site at *http://www.jhbmc.jhu.edu.*

The patient and family information center provides educational materials on many different topics related to heart disease, prevention, and treatment. The main sections are the following:

- Lifestyle—provides information on exercise, nutrition, smoking, and stress, emotion, and behavior modification
- Medical—discusses the pathophysiology of heart disease and related heart health topics
- Heart Health Today—a quarterly newsletter for children and adults that provides tips on the prevention and management of cardiovascular disease, with a focus on lifestyle/behavior changes
- Clinical research studies—announces the research projects in progress
- Links—provides hyperlinks to other patient information and support groups available on the Web

To access the health information sheets (more than 50 different topics are available) and the *Heart Health Today* newsletter, users need to have Adobe Acrobat Reader technology capability. Newsletter archives are available from Spring 1997 to the present. All patient and family educational information as well as the newsletter can be printed for personal use. The site has links to other professional and nonprofessional Web sites that offer relevant information and other resources beneficial to the heart patient. In addition, the site provides search engine capability by topic.

Information available on this site is credible, simple, concise, current, and clear. The date of the last updates made is found on the main page. No site map is available.

MayoClinic.com: Heart and Blood Vessels Center

http://www.mayoclinic.com/home?id=3.1.9

A team of physicians, educators, scientists, and writers directs the Mayo Clinic Web site. The drug companies AstraZenneca, Novartis, and Searle/Pfizer sponsor the site. This site is committed to providing health education to patients, their families, and the general public. An editorial board of Mayo staff identifies important and timely health topics and selects specialists and experts to write about these topics, then publishes this information on the site. The published information remains current and is frequently updated. The site accepts advertising, however, under strict guidelines. For example, no advertisements for promoting alcohol, health/life insurance, or professional medical products are accepted. From the homepage one can access the Heart Center special site. The Heart Center site presents information specific to heart disease.

The features of this site are:

- Headlines—presents news briefs and news alerts
- Ask the Mayo Physician—allows patients and their families to access health information and educational materials. The materials are listed alphabetically to allow easy access. Newly added sources are labeled as such
- Quizzes—allows users to evaluate their knowledge about cholesterol (two quizzes), heart disease (one quiz), and high blood pressure (one quiz). The correct answers to the questions included in the quizzes are provided with further explanation. This feature is a work in progress; more quizzes related to other topics will be added
- Reference Articles—this feature is geared to patient and family education. It presents information similar to a newsletter. Topics are dated and updated to reflect current trends and health care practices
- Life after Sudden Death—people share their personal stories and experiences about heart disease in this section. There are seven stories (or parts, as they are labeled in the site) available to date. In each story, related information about risk factors for heart disease, warning signs for heart attack, and other diagnostic and therapeutic procedures are presented using hyperlinks
- Other Sites—establishes links to related sites, such as the American Heart Association and Mended Hearts Inc. sites (see separate entries)

The site is easy to navigate. It shares reliable information that is simple and clear. The site map on the homepage makes it easy to navigate. This Web site honors the Health on the Net Foundation Code.

A unique feature of this site is the "Interactive Heart Guide," which addresses the pathophysiology of the heart and blood vessels and their associated diseases. This feature is accessible in a simple, attractive, pictorial/text format. Access to the animated format requires Quick Time

Plug-In for Windows technology. Another special feature is *Headline Watch*, an online newsletter published monthly that discusses heart disease and the latest treatments. Previous issues are accessible through the archive menu.

Mended Hearts Inc.

http://www.mendedhearts.org

Mended Hearts Inc. is a nonprofit, all-volunteer organization established in 1951 to provide free educational information and support service for patients suffering from heart disease and their families and caregivers. The site is developed by Jaeger Interactive Media. The 270 volunteer chapters of Mended Hearts are available in 260 cities throughout the United States and Canada. A national board of directors consisting of elected officers, including physicians, nurses, and allied health professionals, governs Mended Hearts and establishes and reinforces its policies. An advisory council, consisting of a group of nationally recognized professionals and citizens, advises and assists the board in the performance of its duties. Currently, Mended Hearts is affiliated with the American Heart Association. A member of the American Association of Critical Care Nurses board of directors serves on the advisory board.

The aims of Mended Hearts are to (1) offer help, support, and encouragement to heart disease patients, their families, and their caregivers; (2) encourage people to deal with the emotional recovery from heart disease; and (3) distribute information of specific educational value. These aims are achieved by visiting patients while in the hospital or at home. Visits are made in person, via the telephone, or through the Internet. The visitors are trained in facilitating emotional recovery, counseling, and offering emotional support. Volunteers of Mended Hearts respond to approximately 3,500 Internet support requests per year. Patients or their families can request the visiting program via the Internet by clicking on the e-mail icon on the homepage.

Other features include:

- Educational information on heart attacks, healthy hearts, and related topics
- Links to other Web sites, including national and international sites as well as online support groups

- Information about hospitals in the United States to help users choose the best place for their care.
- Women and heart disease
- Web links specific to pediatric care

The site is easy to navigate and user-friendly, and the text is written at a lower reading level, which enhances its utility. The resources offered are credible; however, it is difficult to determine if they are current because no dates are available that indicate when the information was posted or last updated. The site does not include a site map, but it is search engine capable.

National Heart, Lung, and Blood Institute: Cardiovascular Information for Patients and the General Public

http://www.nhlbi.nih.gov/health/public/heart/index.htm

The National Heart, Lung, and Blood Institute (NHLBI) is one of the 17 institutes of the National Institutes of Health (NIH). The NIH is a division of the U.S. Department of Health and Human Services. It is the federal government's organization for medical research that aims at enhancing people's health and well-being.

Similar to the Web sites of the other institutes, the NHLBI site includes a health information section that is divided into two categories, one for patients and the general public and the other for health care professionals. Consumer-related information is available under the patients and general public category. Users can access different types of information in this category, such as:

- High blood pressure—presents patient educational materials specific to high blood pressure control and prevention. It also includes information about the National High Blood Pressure Education Program, which is a program of professional, patient, and public education available to reduce death and disability related to high blood pressure
- Cholesterol—shares facts about cholesterol and eating healthy and tips for lowering cholesterol blood level. It also includes information about the National Cholesterol Education Program, which aims to raise awareness about cholesterol as a risk factor for coronary heart disease
- Obesity—discusses healthy weight, physical activity, calculating body mass index, and facts about heart disease and women. It

also includes information about the Obesity Education Initiative, which aims to reduce the prevalence of obesity and enhance physical activity
* Heart attack—raises awareness of warning signs for heart attack, encourages timely access to medical attention, discusses the risk factors for heart disease, and shares strategies for preventing prehospital treatment delays for myocardial infarction
* Other cardiovascular topics—includes information and fact sheets about various cardiovascular diseases and how this information can be purchased in bulk amount. Users can obtain single copies free of charge. Requests can be made online, via telephone using a toll-free number, or through the mail
* Latino cardiovascular health resources—features patient and family educational materials that are available in Spanish. Such information is in booklet format and can be obtained free of charge in single copies

The information shared on this site is clear, concise, and simple. Users can navigate the site easily. Some of the information requires Acrobat Reader or Java Script capability for downloading or printing. Of all the sites reviewed in this chapter, this is the only one that provides information on normal and age-specific values of blood pressure, cholesterol, weight, and heart rate. It also describes exercise programs, exercise recommendations, and number of calories based on type of exercise. However, it is difficult to determine whether this information is current because no dates are provided to indicate when the information was posted online or last updated.

A unique feature of this site is the Healthbeat Radio Program, which sponsors a 60-second heart health information tip on 500 radio stations nationwide. These information bites are available on the site in audio format. Users can listen to them using Real Player technology. Other features of this site are links to other Web sites and search capability. The search engine is specific to the NIH site; that is, the search is completed across all 17 institutes. Users can search by topic, word, or phrase. Search tips are also available to enhance results.

REFERENCE

Centers for Disease Control and Prevention. (2000). Preventing cardiovascular disease: Addressing the nation's leading killer, at-a-glance 2000. [Online]. Accessed on October 24, 2000, *http://www.cdc.gov/nccdphp/cvd/cvdaag.htm*.

Chapter 20

HIV/AIDS

Carl A. Kirton, MA, RN, ANP-CS, ACRN and
Joseph P. Colagreco, MS, RN, ANP-CS

This chapter highlights several HIV/AIDS Web sites that can be used as adjuncts to health information provided by health care professionals. These sites were chosen based on several attributes:

1. Timeliness: Although major changes in the treatment of HIV have slowed, small changes continue to occur. Sites that reflect only the latest changes in HIV information were chosen.
2. Readability: The average HIV-infected adult may not be familiar with medical or technical jargon. Sites were chosen that would appeal to readers of various reading levels and levels of HIV sophistication.
3. Broadness: HIV demographics are vast; therefore, sites were chosen that would appeal to all types of HIV-infected individuals—women, men, gay, newly diagnosed, or HIV experienced.
4. Overall appeal: We asked ourselves, "Would I want my patient reading this site?"

AIDS Action

http://www.aidsaction.org

Founded in 1984, AIDS Action is the only organization solely dedicated to responsible federal policy for improved HIV/AIDS care and services, vigorous medical research, and effective prevention. The site is impressively designed, but because of its design the graphics take a long time to download. Yet some of the design elements don't seem to fit the rest of the site. For example, the virtual vaccine link engenders a multimedia experience, only to give rise to more text with a black background, which is markedly different from any other page on this site.

One of the impressive elements of this site is the authors' recognition that not all readers are at the same level of knowledge with respect to policy issues. To meet the needs of all readers, the authors have organized content into three levels. For each issue, the reader chooses the level that best fits his or her needs. The green circle icon directs beginners, the blue square ushers intermediate-level readers to content, and the black diamond jettisons the expert to appropriate content areas.

AIDS Education Global Information System (AEGIS)

http://www.aegis.org

The purpose of this site is to disseminate AEGIS information. AEGIS is the largest online HIV/AIDS knowledge base in the world, with more than 341,000 files on its server, including, but not limited to, the National Library of Medicine's AIDSDRUGS, AIDSLINE, and AIDSTRIALS. The site claims that the information is updated hourly.

Unique to this site is the "Law Library," where U.S. court decisions and law-oriented journals related to HIV/AIDS are available.

Although this site is for the sophisticated consumer of HIV information, almost anyone who wants any reading material from popular magazines to professional literature will find it here.

AIDSmeds.com

http://www.aidsmeds.com

The mission of *AIDSmeds.com* is to provide people living with HIV the necessary information they need to make empowered treatment decisions. The site claims to offer complete, but not complicated, up-to-date information.

The site is full of "lessons" that offer the reader simplified information to questions such as "What are T cells?" and "When should I start treatment?" Definitions for almost all medical terms and drugs appear in "pop-up" boxes when users click on words they don't know. On pages where there are medical news stories there is a call box titled "What's That Mean?" By typing in the word, the user can learn the definition.

Other features of the site are the patient's ability to build a medication list with pertinent drug information and the lifelike laboratory reports. There is a page with all of the approved drugs listed, with adult dosages, side effects, and any special notes. The pictures of the drugs, however, are difficult to see.

The site is for the sophisticated computer user. The typeface is small and can be difficult to read. The advertising banners are large and distracting. This overwhelming advertising deters a solid endorsement of the site.

The Body: An AIDS and HIV Information Resource

http://www.thebody.com

The Body's mission "is to use the Web to lower barriers between patients and clinicians, demystify HIV/AIDS and its treatment, improve patients' quality of life, [and] foster community through human connection." Patients directed to this site will find there are more than 250 topic areas covering almost every aspect of HIV/AIDS. The Body is produced by Body Health Resources Corp. of New York. It has many commercial drug firms as sponsors.

The site provides excellent reprints of articles on understanding HIV, working with a doctor, first steps to treatment, telling others, and women-specific treatment issues. This feature might be improved if the articles were full-text PDF files.

Professional conference coverage is excellent. It is written in language that can be understood by almost any level of reader.

Patients can submit questions to an expert panel of clinicians (you even get to see a picture of the expert to whom you submit your question). The responses are short, simple, and factual.

Unique to this site is the "Visual AIDS Web Gallery." It comprises works selected from the Visual AIDS' Archive Project. The gallery exhibitions change every 6 weeks.

This Web site contains a link to *POZ* magazine, a popular lay publication that is concerned with HIV/AIDS. This link indicates a sensitivity to community-based information. Another indication of community sensitivity is the availability of this site in Spanish—with a simple click.

Overall, this is an important site for anyone wishing to access HIV/AIDS information.

CDC Guide to Caring for Someone with AIDS at Home

http://www.hivatis.org/caring

This site provides basic information about HIV—how to give care, protect against infections, recognize symptoms, make decisions, and provide emotional support. It is an excellent resource for someone with a loved one or a family member who is cared for at home with HIV. The most unfortunate thing about this site is that the text cannot be printed in a more user-friendly format. Also of note is that the typeface is large and the reading level is low. Although the sophisticated reader might take issue with the large typeface and low reading level, these are advantages in getting the information to the widest possible audience. In fact, this site should be required reading for those with someone at home with HIV. The site is sponsored by the U.S. Centers for Disease Control and Prevention.

HIV InSite

http://www.hivinsite.ucsf.edu

This site, sponsored by the University of California, San Francisco, covers HIV/AIDS treatment, policy, research, prevention, statistics, and epidemiology. It is geared for professionals, but consumers will also find this an excellent source of information.

The site gives the latest information on treatment recommendations. It includes citations from various clinical and government agencies. As an added feature, *The AIDS Knowledge Base*, 1999 edition, by P. T. Cohen, Merle A. Sande, and Paul A. Volberding, is available free online (the 1994 edition is also available). Another special feature is expert clinician advice and consultation online. There is also the equivalent of a "virtual book club"; visit the site regularly for slides and audio lectures from experts in the field. If you can have only HIV/AIDS Web site, this is it.

The content of the site is extremely accurate and useful. The site is well maintained, with a user-friendly interface.

National Association on HIV Over 50

http://www.hivoverfifty.org

See review in Chapter 14, "Elders and Their Families."

Pets Are Loving Support

http://www.sonic.net/~pals

Sometimes people with HIV want a break from learning about treatment and laboratory data. The above site is hosted by a nonprofit agency "organized to improve the quality of life of people with AIDS by preserving and promoting the human/animal bond through the care and maintenance of their animal companions."

Recently redesigned and still under construction, the site may be time consuming to download. Nevertheless, the authors address important issues such as pet hygiene, veterinary care, and animal bites.

Once the problems are resolved, this may become an important site to anyone with HIV who owns a pet.

Pregnancy and HIV

http://www.hcfa.gov/hiv

See review in Chapter 27, "Pregnancy and Childbirth."

The Yoga Group: Yoga for HIV/AIDS

http://www.yogagroup.org

Another site that may be of interest to those with HIV is that sponsored by The Yoga Group, a Colorado nonprofit organization providing free yoga classes and information since 1988 to persons living with HIV/AIDS. The site can help other yoga teachers start similar programs.

Youth Resource

http://www.youthresource.com

It appears that young adults with HIV must find their support at adult sites. Sadly, there is a paucity of HIV/AIDS-dedicated sites for teens with HIV.

Most HIV youth sites are intervention projects attached to a major university or a study project that has a prevention focus. Although prevention is important, young adults with HIV need their own special forum.

Youth Resource is directed primarily toward the gay, lesbian, and transgendered youth. This site has links to other HIV/AIDS sites, most dealing with preventing teen HIV. There are links to other sites profiling teens living with HIV. There are also links to pages for youths dealing with sexually transmitted diseases. Unfortunately, a visit to some of these sites quickly demonstrates that not all pages are of value.

The site "feels" like a page written by youths for youths rather than a university- or community-based project; as such, it is more likely to appeal to young people.

Chapter 21

Immunization and Screening

Linda Peters, MS, RN, CPNP

The Web sites selected here all offer an overview and easy explanation of current vaccinations for childhood diseases. In addition, some sites offer information on the current disease status and immunizations requirements for travelers throughout the world. For more information on travelers' health, see Chapter 34, "Travel Considerations." Parental and professional misconceptions are addressed in the following Web sites, using objective data. Risks for delaying immunizations are covered. The sites listed provide a comprehensive yet concise reference for parents.

Babycenter—Immunizations: What You Need to Know About Them

http://www.babycenter.com/refcap/95.html

This site offers a commonsense explanation of vaccines using a question-and-answer format. Experts from Babycenter describe how vaccines work, as well as their safety and efficacy. Included is a one-sentence description of the eight most common immunizations. Babycenter is sponsored by Johnson & Johnson. It provides information and products to new and expecting parents.

Information is accurate and updated. A unique section titled "Polls and Debates" offers tips and viewpoints from parenting peers, thus encouraging sharing. Information is available on 38 related subtopics, from the risks of delaying vaccinations to where vaccinations can be obtained at low cost. The site is visually appealing and interesting. Information is limited to ages 0 to 24 months. However, a link to Parentcenter gives information on 2- to 8-year-olds. Text is in English only.

Dr. Greene's Housecalls

http://www.drgreene.com/immunizations.asp

This site, which provides practical information on the most common issues regarding immunization, features questions answered by a caring, perceptive pediatrician, Alan Greene, MD, FAAP. Dr. Greene is cofounder of *Adam.com*, a commercial health information Web site. Parents will find this site useful because the questions come from other concerned parents.

Information is reliable and accurate. The overview includes an interesting history, a description of current practices and research, and a list of risks and benefits. Information is given in a friendly, nonthreatening manner. The site is learner-friendly and less wordy than other sites. A weak point is that it is not culturally sensitive.

Immunizations: What You Need to Know

http://www.aap.org/family/vaccine.htm

The American Academy of Pediatrics, which sponsors this site, offers an informative explanation of the usefulness and the necessity of childhood vaccines. The site clears up misunderstandings parents have regarding immunizations by providing rational explanations using a no-nonsense approach. Parents are the intended audience. Information is current and accurate.

The site addresses issues that are often not found on other sites, such as the need for immunizations for breastfed babies, the need for vaccinations for diseases that are no longer common, and how to deal with the pain of an injection. A brief description of the role of the U.S. Food and Drug Administration is helpful. Communication with health care providers is encouraged and empowers parents to work with physicians by outlining the parents' responsibilities. Information is easy to understand. Brief explanations of common misconceptions make this site useful and practical.

What Would Happen If We Stopped Vaccinations?

http://www.cdc.gov/nip/publications/fs/gen/WhatIfStop.htm

This site provides an overview of the impact of vaccine-preventable diseases. Its purpose is to outline the morbidity and mortality of disease on the individual family, the country, and the world. It is produced by the Centers for Disease Control. Parents and health care providers are the intended audience.

Information is current and accurate. The site lists the incidence of each of the most common childhood diseases in the world and how that would change if vaccinations were stopped. The presentation is factual and objective, brief, and to the point.

Chapter 22

Incontinence—Urinary and Bowel

Sandra Jones, MA, RN and Audrey J. Schmerzler, MSN, RN, CRRN

Incontinence is a condition that affects millions of Americans. Although it is commonly thought to be a disorder of the elderly, it can actually occur in early and middle adulthood as well. This condition leads to emotional distress, physical discomfort, and social isolation. Incontinence is not a normal condition of aging and often can be controlled to enhance the quality of life. The following Web sites can help those dealing with incontinence to understand the problem and to provide guidance for diagnosis and treatment. The sites should be used along with guidance from a health care provider.

URINARY INCONTINENCE
Reviewer: Sandra Jones, MA, RN

American Foundation for Urologic Disease

http://www.afud.org
(Click on "Urological Diseases," then "Diseases and Conditions," then click on "Incontinence")

The site is sponsored by the American Foundation for Urologic Disease and is written for consumers. There is no date indicating the currency of the content, but information is consistent with current literature and practice. The text is written only in English.

Users will find descriptions of incontinence, statistics, causes and types of incontinence (stress, urge, mixed, functional, nocturnal eneuresis), diagnostic tests (urinalysis, postvoid residual catheterization, ultrasound, cystoscopy, urodynamic testing), and treatment modalities. There is a short quiz at the end, and answers can be submitted by e-mail for evaluation.

This is an excellent site that is easy to read. It combines text with bulleted lists. Several terms are underlined and colored to provide links to either a glossary or diagrams. The site also includes a bladder diary form that patients can use before seeing a physician or while in treatment.

One weakness is found in the section on treatment. Modalities are listed and briefly explained, but there is no description of behavioral modifications or pelvic floor exercises.

The site is very easy to navigate. Sections can be accessed by clicking on the options at the bottom of each section.

Bladder Control for Women

http://www.niddk.nih.gov
(Click on "urologic," "incontinence," then title)

or *http://www.niddk.nih.gov/health/urolog/uibcw/index.htm*

Sponsored by the National Institute of Diabetes, Digestive, and Kidney Disorders (NIDDK), a division of the National Institutes of Health, the site addresses why incontinence is an issue, where to get help, information to take to the doctor (including a bladder diary), usual diagnostic tests, causes of incontinence, and treatment. The treatment section addresses lifestyle, pelvic exercises, muscle therapy, devices, medications, surgery, and dryness aids.

The strength of the site is its easy-to-read, well-organized format that includes graphics and bulleted lists. The information is thorough, and there are addresses for additional sources. There are also links to more detailed publications available through the NIDDK.

There are no major weaknesses. Although the text is simply written, it is long, which can be difficult for weak readers. This site also requires the use of Adobe Acrobat reader. The site is also available in Spanish.

Facts About Incontinence

http://www.nafc.org

Sponsored by the National Association for Continence and written for consumers, the site provides a brief overview of incontinence, as well as links to additional literature, products, and services available for people experiencing incontinence. The site defines five types of incontinence, describes the causes and treatment options, and advises users to seek professional help. Visitors to the site can learn the warning signs of incontinence, the steps to take, and the information needed when seeking assistance.

The strength of the site is its encouragement and direction to seek medical help and its links to products and services. Its weakness is the information provided. Although the content is valid, the information is very general, with minimal detail. The links to literature require the purchase of the materials.

The site is easy to navigate, simply written, and available in English only.

Urinary Incontinence: Embarrassing but Treatable

http://www.familydoctor.org/healthfacts/189/index.html

This site is designed for consumers and is sponsored by the American Academy of Family Physicians. It is divided into five sections addressing the definitions of three types of incontinence (stress, urge, and overflow), causes, relationship to aging, and treatment modalities. The information is consistent with current literature and practice.

Information is well organized, and the text is simply written. There are brief directions for pelvic floor exercises that are presented in a table format. This is a good resource to use as an introduction to incontinence. The very simple language allows this site to be used for individuals with low reading skills.

The main weakness is its brevity. A discussion of medication therapy is brief and incomplete, citing only the use of topical estrogen. There is very little detail and will require additional support from health care providers and/or other literature. The print is also very small.

The site is easy to navigate. At the homepage, type in "incontinence" and click on "search." Each section is clearly listed and can be accessed separately. The "Family Doctor" homepage allows consumers to type in and access several topics easily.

NEUROGENIC BOWEL INCONTINENCE

Reviewer: Audrey J. Schmerzler, RN, MSN, RNC

It was extremely difficult to find this topic on the Net. There was no site devoted exclusively to neurogenic bowel incontinence. Rather, this topic was a section in other Web sites, usually sites devoted to a specific disease or disability. Few of the sites were targeted to consumers; several were aimed at educators who may have children with disabilities in their classes, and only a few were devoted to health care professionals.

Neurogenic Bowel Management in Adults with Spinal Cord Injury

Http://www.pva.org/pubsandproducts/pvapubs/BowelProfessional.htm

and

Neurogenic Bowel: What You Should Know

http://www.pva.org/sci/pubs/consumerbowelmain.htm

The Paralyzed Veterans of America (PVA) has a large Web site geared toward consumers, in particular, veterans with spinal cord injuries. One of its missions has been to develop clinical practice guidelines (CPG) to educate and instruct professionals in certain aspects of care. In addition to CPGs, three accompanying consumer guidelines have been published. Regarding neurogenic bowel incontinence, both the CPGs and the consumer guidelines are well written, easy to understand (for the intended audience), and extremely informative. The CPGs for professionals are thorough and cover all aspects of neurogenic bowel incontinence, from a summary of recommendations to an algorithm of designing an effective bowel program, to a list of references. The consumer guide is less detailed but just as effective. The language is easy to understand; illustrations are provided to emphasize points. The text can be downloaded, or a hard copy can be purchased.

The one criticism of the main site (*http://www.pva.org*) where the above two guidelines can be found is that the guidelines are hard to locate. However, the site is in the process of being redesigned for easier access and use.

Most of the rehabilitation hospital sites are linked to the PVA site.

Taking Care of Your Bowels: The Basics

http://www.djepson.wiredup.com/bowel1.html

This Web site gives a basic overview of neurogenic bowel incontinence. It covers all aspects of a fundamental bowel routine but does not go into any great depth. The intended audience is newly injured people with spinal cord injuries and their significant others. It is sponsored by Harborview Medical Center, Rehabilitation Medicine Clinic, Seattle, WA, and is part of a larger educational site sponsored by Harborview.

Chapter 23

Infertility

Nancy E. Reame, PhD, RN, FAAN

nfertility is a problem that plagues a growing number of couples eager to have children, many of them trying to start a family in midlife. Infertility makes some potential parents desperate to seek a solution and has become a big business. There are many doctors who make a substantial profit by helping couples to conceive, whether or not the couples ever manage to have children. The following Web site was chosen because it is a patient advocacy organization and seemed least biased toward the "business" of solving infertility.

RESOLVE: The National Infertility Association

http://www.resolve.org

RESOLVE: the National Infertility Association is the premier patient advocacy association founded in 1974 by nurse Barbara Menning to provide information and support for individuals experiencing infertility. Its Web site presents not only basic medical information about infertility treatments but also policy positions, regular summaries of current legislation and clinical trials, press releases, a bulletin board, a bookstore, and an advocacy update e-mail service. Links to other resources include local chapters, a national help line, and the important annual national status report from the Centers for Disease Control regarding infertility clinic practices and success rates. Some areas of the site, such as the quarterly newsletter and physician referral list, are open only to members. A disclaimer page warns visitors that RESOLVE does not endorse or recommend the infertility specialists featured in the referral list, nor does it guarantee the accuracy of information provided by its Web site sponsors. However, given its nonprofit status, its need for financial support, and the cut-throat competition that dominates the infertility specialty, it is not surprising that the majority of site sponsors are the large pharmaceutical manufacturers of fertility medications, as well as the clinic entrepreneurs whose thinly veiled advertising banners are somewhat annoying. As with all bulletin board/ chat room resources, consumers should be aware that not all information is accurate or relevant to their specific situation when it comes to advice from other patients about medications, treatment responses, and help with managing the emotional turmoil of the infertility experience. A better strategy for advice seeking would be to access the "Questions to Ask" fact sheets prepared by RESOLVE on a variety of topics to help consumers navigate the infertility health care industry. Those on buying medications over the Internet and finding an infertility specialist are especially good. Given the numerous and complex medical and social issues involved in infertility management, this user-friendly Web site provides a high level of useful information for both the first-time patient and the seasoned veteran struggling with life-transforming decisions in family building through assisted reproduction, adoption, or child-free living.

Chapter 24

Mental Health

Devon Berry, MSN, RN

M ental health is quickly moving toward the top of the list of the world's major health problems. Although many efforts have been made at both the local and national levels to deal with the growing problem, quality, cost, and access continue to be major barriers to individuals and families in need of care. The Internet represents one possibility of reducing the barriers that currently exist. As the "digital divide" shrinks and the utilization of the Internet becomes more of a societal norm, health care providers will have increasing opportunity to direct their clients to the Internet for help. In this chapter, several Web sites are presented to which health care professionals can confidently direct their clients.

Internet Mental Health

http://www.mentalhealth.com/p.html

Internet Mental Health is a "free encyclopedia of mental health information" that provides users with access to multilingual information on the description, diagnosis, and treatment of mental illnesses. Also given are research studies, information booklets, and magazine articles for over 50 of the most common mental health disorders. The impetus for this site grew originally from a mental health information exchange between Japanese and Canadian mental health professionals. The Canadian contingent developed the Internet site to make a large body of information on mental health disorders easily accessible.

This site, originating in 1995, has been developed and updated by Phillip W. Long, MD, a Canadian psychiatrist, and programmed by Brian Chow. The site has no corporate or institutional sponsors and is completely funded by Dr. Long. This site targets consumers of mental health care and their friends and families, mental health professionals, students, and the general public.

The information presented is up-to-date, relevant to consumers, informative, and accurate. The site has been organized into several main content areas, including description, diagnosis, treatment, and research. There is also a "magazine" area that provides either external or internal links to both scholarly and lay publications on multiple disorders. Numerous links are also provided. These links, however, are not reviewed or necessarily endorsed by the author.

Overall, the site is valuable for several reasons. First, it is not corporate funded. That fact can alleviate a good deal of concern as to the bias of information. Second, the span of information available at the site is comprehensive, and all information, whether from internal or external sources, is provided within the frame of Internet Mental Health. This means that users need never leave the site, which is convenient for both inexperienced and experienced Web browsers. Finally, the site has several unique features, including automated algorithmic diagnostic tools of all the major disorders and availability in six languages.

Mental Help Net

http://mentalhelp.net

Mental Help Net touts itself as being the "oldest and largest online mental health guide and community." It acts as both a hub, organizing and rating many other external links, and a central source of information.

The authors of this site seek to optimize the utilization of online communication to educate the public about mental health issues; help coordinate various components of the mental health field; catalog, review, and make available to everyone all online mental health resources as they become available; and improve access to mental health services and information about mental health services. Although this list is not exhaustive, it accurately communicates the value of this site for the consumer.

This site is sponsored by CMHC Systems and is directed by Mark Dombeck, PhD. CMHC is a provider of information technology for health care and human services. Mental Help Net accepts advertising and sponsorships. It does not make a clear statement as to its audience; however, there are parts of the site that can greatly benefit consumers. There are also many areas from which professionals would benefit.

The information on this site is usually research-based, comprehensive, and written at a level that could be understood by many persons without training in the area of mental health. Under each disorder, the reader is provided with information on and links to symptoms, treatment, research, online resources, organizations, and online support. This makes the site especially valuable.

It is also impressive that the authors of the content at this site are careful to discriminate between what is popularly believed and what is supported by research. A further feature of this site is the rating system it employs. Because there are so many mental health sites on the Internet, it is often helpful to have a dependable source that rates and ranks the quality of the sites.

Mentalwellness.com: The Online Resource for Schizophrenia and Other Mental Health Information

http://www.mentalwellness.com

Mentalwellness.com is a good example of a genre of mental health Web sites focused on providing support versus information. The titles of some of the areas in this site include "Help Is at Hand," "Feature Stories," "Help and Hope," and "Behind the Mask." There is also some very practical information at this site, including "Dollars and Sense," which includes articles providing simple advice on sound money management principles, and "Reference Room," which provides information on common mental health disorders, mental health links, and recommended readings.

This site is both sponsored and controlled by Janssen Pharmaceutica Products LP and is clearly designed with the consumer in mind. Its design is clean, simple, and easy to navigate. The material at this site is well written, clear, and generally very encouraging to the person experiencing a mental illness. As intended, it is foreseeable that users of this site could develop a sense of community, understanding, and hope secondary to browsing its many resources.

National Institute of Mental Health

Http://www.nimh.nih.gov

The National Institute of Mental Health (NIMH) has long had an interest in serving the needs of the mental health population and continues to do so through the "For the Public" section of its Web page. This section offers information from the NIMH about the symptoms, diagnosis, and treatment of mental illnesses. Included are brochures and information sheets, reports, press releases, fact sheets, and other educational materials. It also provides a variety of information in Spanish. The NIMH acts as the funding source for this site and claims responsibility for all content and information.

The material available at this site is outstanding in most cases. Information is written at a level accessible to most and is clear and accurate. The information is research-based and regularly updated. Often the articles are provided in PDF format, which resolves any formatting issues and makes printing exceptionally easy. This site can be a great resource for information for both consumers and practitioners in mental health; however, it should not be considered a strong resource for consumers seeking psychosocial support in their experience of a mental health disorder.

Stayhealthy.com

http://www.stayhealthy.com

Stayhealthy.com is a broad, comprehensive site encouraging people to take control of their health. It seeks to accomplish this goal by creating "tools of empowerment." Although this site is valuable in many ways, its drug information program can be especially helpful to consumers.

Stayhealthy Inc. is a privately held corporation based in Iowa and California. Dr. Colin Hill, director of biomedical information at Stayhealthy Inc. and associate professor of radiation oncology and molecular microbiology at the University of Southern California Norris Cancer Center, works with a medical advisory board to approve all content and information. *Stayhealthy.com* has been designed with consumers in mind and is therefore very browser-friendly.

Among the many drug reference sites available on the Internet, this one stands out for several reasons. First, it is easy to navigate. The site is arranged simply, and the absence of flashing ads reduces distractions. Second, the information provided is clear and accurate and written for the consumer. Each information sheet includes the generic name, dosage, route, common uses (vs. indicated), cautions, possible side effects, and additional information. A clear and up-close picture of the actual medication is also provided for some drugs. Third, the information generally prints out on one page. Finally, for the consumer desiring more in-depth information, several links are often given for further information with each drug. Because mental health consumers are often very curious about their medication and its effects, an easy-to-use drug reference Web site can be very helpful.

Chapter 25

Neurological Problems

Graham J. McDougall, Jr., PhD, RN, CS

N eurological problems can take many forms, ranging from multiple sclerosis and Parkinson's disease to a simple headache. This chapter reviews three megasites for neurological disorders. The final review is a specialty site covering headaches, which afflict more individuals than any other neurological problem.

Disability-Specific Web Site

http://www.disserv.stu.umn.edu/disability

This megasite gives 159 hyperlinks to other neurological Web sites. The sites are listed alphabetically, from "Americans with Disabilities Act" to "wheelchair carriers." No information on sponsorship was available.

Global Neurologic Web Sites

http://www.neuro.onnet.co.kr/links.html

This megasite has hyperlinks to 800 Web sites. This site is organized by diseases, symptoms, and academic research centers. Classifications are neurology/neuroscience news, associations/societies, neurology/neuroscience departments, cerebrovascular accident, epilepsy, headache, dementia—Alzheimer's disease, intracranial neoplasm,

multiple sclerosis, motor neuron disease (ALS), movement disorder—
Parkinson's disease, infectious disease, spinal cord disease, myasthe-
nia gravis, peripheral nerve disease, muscle disease, sleep disorder,
vertigo/dizziness, development disease, neuro-ophthalmology, pediatric neurology, neuroscience, Atlas-Gross, Micropathology, books/arti-
cles, and other worthwhile sites. This site is part of Han NeuroNet, a
collaboration between Keimyung University's Dongsan Medical Center
in South Korea and physician Yong Won Cho.

National Headache Foundation

http://www.headaches.org

The National Headache Foundation (NHF), a nonprofit organization,
sponsors this site, and identifies Suzanne E. Simons as the Executive
Director and Seymour Diamond, MD as the Executive Chairman. The
three-fold mission is inform, research, and educate. The site advertises
itself as "Your #1 Source for Headache Help." The site offers consumer
information on specific headache conditions and treatments, educational materials for purchase, information about headache support
groups, and excerpts from the NHF's *Head Lines*. Features include a
full-text publication of the *Complete Guide to Headache*, a national
listing of support groups available in 23 states, and 10 steps for migraine
sufferers. Other relevant topics include myths of caffeine and headaches and children's headaches. The site has hyperlinks to 10 pharmaceutical companies that make products to treat headaches.The most
interesting aspect of the site is IMPACT, a six-step self-help process
for migraine sufferers. The steps are to 1) Identify the symptoms of
migraine; 2) Maintain a diary of your migraine history; 3) Proactively
partner with your health care provider; 4) Avoid situations that cause
migraines; 5) Contact the National Headache Foundation; and 6) Treat
your migraine effectively. A headache diary is available online and is
clearly laid out so that an individual can begin immediately to identify
the date, time, intensity rating, preceding symptoms, triggers, medication, and relief.

Even though a separate page is listed for clinical trials, at the time
of this review none were listed. The site is pleasing to the eye and
easy to navigate, and provides information that is immediately useful
to the consumer.

See also Chapter 33 on Stroke.

National Institute of Neurological Disorders and Stroke

http://www.ninds.nih.gov

This easy-to-navigate site gives information on funding and recent news related to important scientific findings. Two sections are highlighted. The "Browse All Disorders" section consists of 204 neurological conditions arranged alphabetically. Each condition lists the description, treatment, prognosis, research, references, and organizations associated with the particular disorder. The "Organizations" section, arranged alphabetically, provides hyperlinks to patient resources, foundations, and supportive organizations. In addition, the consumer may request free brochures. NINDS is sponsored by the U.S. government.

Chapter 26

Pain

Laree J. Schoolmeesters, MSN, RN

Pain is a common experience among all people. Nurses need to know how to provide support and information to individuals experiencing pain. The following Web sites introduce readers to the education resources available on the Net. Factual information on pain and its treatment can be found on the American Academy of Pain Management, Mayday Pain Project, Pediatric Pain, and Talarian Index Web sites. For those who need assistance in communicating their pain experience, see the Infomin, Pain.com, and Pediatric Pain sites. Infomin and Pain.com are ideal for chronic pain sufferers who feel isolated and alone in their pain experience. For nurses looking for continuing education credit, stop in at Pain.com. Use all of these sites to help end needless suffering.

American Academy of Pain Management

http://www.aapainmanage.org

The American Academy of Pain Management (AAPM) is a multidisciplinary pain society that provides credentialing for board certification in pain management. The site is intended for physicians. It provides information about AAPM membership, the congressional record, and continuing medical education. The site provides a number of beneficial resources for consumers. These include guides to U.S. pain management programs and professionals, organized by zip code, the Patients'

Bill of Rights, pain management definitions, and related links. The related links provide access to resources, associations, comprehensive information sites, medical institutions, government resources, pain research, clinics, pain publications, and e-zines. This site's most valuable feature is the up-to-date and accurate National Pain Data Bank, which allows searches to be performed pairing a pain condition with treatments or medications. The text is in English and written at an average to high-average reading level. The site is easy to navigate.

InfoMIN: Medical Information Network for Chronic Pain, CFS, FMS, and Other Medical Resources

http://www2.rpa.net/~lrandall/index.html

InfoMIN is a private, nonprofit health information resource, maintained by Lois Randall, a chronic pain sufferer, that offers medical information for patients, family members, and health care providers. The current information covers numerous topics, such as chronic pain, chronic fatigue syndrome (CFS), fibromyalgia, reflex sympathetic dystrophy, myofascial pain syndrome, Crohn's disease, and depression and chronic illness. The site uses large fonts and provides information on how to obtain Social Security Disability and about pain policy and law for the disabled. Both health care providers and consumers can use the "Pain Inventory Form" and "Pain Diary Worksheet," which are downloadable.

The text, in English only, covers a wide variety of chronic pain disorders. Links are given to mainstream medical sources as well as complementary therapy sites. Included with each link is a synopsis, as well as related articles, support groups, and university-based research projects.

InfoMIN is an excellent, frequently updated resource for nurses, patients, and family members. Its weaknesses are the repetitiveness of some of the material and the fact that lay opinions are included. Yet this very weakness is a bond that pain patients will appreciate, giving insight into their own experiences and feelings.

Mayday Pain Project

http://www.painandhealth.org

The purpose of the Mayday Pain Project is to increase awareness of and provide objective information concerning the treatment of pain.

This Web site is an index for visitors and contains carefully chosen Internet links and resources. The site is designed for pain sufferers, family members, caregivers, and medical professionals. It is sponsored by the Mayday Fund, a philanthropic fund dedicated to alleviating pain.

The site has two major headings: "Internet Resources" and "Health News." The best feature is "Internet Resources." Subheadings include specific pain-producing diseases (e.g., arthritis), general pain, pain and depression, senior pain, pharmacology, hospitals and therapies, and journals and periodicals. Each subheading has an alphabetical list of Internet sites, organizations, and articles, followed by a brief description about the sites. Some subheadings list helpful top 10 sites. The "Health News" section contains information on continuing medical education, living with pain, and confidential pain surveys.

One weakness is a lack of information provided by the pain project itself, which seems to be limited to a brief introduction to the Internet subheadings and the living with pain link. A second weakness would be the lack of more top ten sites. The site provides information in English and is simple to use with newly added Internet sites located on the home page.

Pain.com

http://www.pain.com

Pain.com is funded by the Dannemiller Memorial Educational Foundation and identifies resources for consumers and health care professionals. Features include a glossary, a list of support groups, a helpful advice column written by a chronic pain sufferer, and printable pain assessment forms that can be used to communicate with physicians. A free service is "Ask the Pain Doctor," with replies sent to a message board. Other resources are international organizations, health newsstand, pain publications, pain studies, and libraries. A link to a drug checker is available to determine any medication or food interaction. Links are given to pain studies, libraries, and policy reports. Nurses will appreciate the free Continuing Medical Education credit with certificates that can be printed from the computer, information from the World Health Organization Collaborating Center for Policy and Communications in Cancer Care, and JCAHO (Joint Commission on Accreditation of Health Care Organizations) pain standards. A new feature is expert physician interviews regarding pain topics. The *Online Pain Journal* is exceptional, with entire text and references available to read and print.

Consumers and nurses will benefit from the extensive virtual library, with almost 4,000 articles from abstracts, case studies, and journals. Searches may be done using author, keywords, or title. This site is current, comprehensive, well designed, and visually appealing. The information is in English and is easily accessible.

Pediatric Pain

http://is.dal.ca/%7Epedpain/pedpain.html

The Psychology Department of Dalhousie University in Canada and the IWK Grace Health Center run a pediatric pain research laboratory that provides professional, research, pediatric pain, and self-help resources, each with related links. Nurses can explore the "International Forum on Pediatric Pain," which focuses on cutting-edge research and clinical practice, and the "Child Facial Coding Scale," a behavioral coding system to estimate a child's pain. Other resources are the "Pediatric Pain Letter," containing abstracts and commentaries, and the "Mailing List," which is an international forum for discussion about children's pain. The Pediatric Pain source book of protocol policies and pamphlets can be downloaded onto a disk. The source book can be searched based on keywords in the areas of audience (e.g., children, parents), pain type, drug type, nonpharmacological method, disease, and more. This information is at a high reading level.

The self-help section is easy for both parents and nurses to use. Two online booklets are available in English. *Pain, Pain Go Away: Helping Children with Pain* is illustrated with suggestions for pain relief and is written at an above-average reading level. *Making Cancer Less Painful: A Handbook for Parents* discusses the potential pain involved with cancer and surgical procedures. Pediatric Pain links are listed alphabetically, detailing organizations and self-help sites, including pain management and financial resources for children and parents. This is an excellent, well-rounded site that gives current research-based information.

The Talarian Index

http://www.stat.washington.edu/TALARIA/talaria0/TALARIA.html

This site, maintained by David Madigan and Ying Zhang, offers hypermedia clinical practice guidelines for cancer pain, although the site covers a broad spectrum of pain definitions. The site is intended for health care professionals, yet consumers would find the index straight-forward and simple to use. The Talarian Index is an alphabetical listing in English of various types of pain, medications, surgery, treatments, and patient education. Just click on a topic of interest and find the information formatted as text, glossary, tables, figures, attachments, and movies. Much of the information is provided with current refer-ences. Related sites have links to well-known information about pain, cancer, and other sources. This site is an up-to-date and accurate pain resource. The best feature is its simplicity; its weakness is its lack of in-depth information on any one topic.

Chapter 27

Pregnancy and Childbirth

Kristen S. Montgomery, PhD, RNC, IBCLC

Women embarking on pregnancy for the first time often have many questions relating to the normal changes of pregnancy, what to expect during labor and delivery, and caring for their newborn. Most pregnancies in the United States are unplanned; therefore, the majority of women who become pregnant in any given year are not very knowledgeable regarding the reproductive cycle, and many of them suddenly find themselves unprepared to cope with the demands of pregnancy. The following Web sites gives helpful, accurate information on pregnancy and childbirth.

BirthPlan.com

http://www.birthplan.com

BirthPlan.com is an interactive birth planning tool that provides parents with information and choices to consider regarding birth. The purpose is to make women and their families aware of what options they have during the birth process. The site is sponsored by *Parenting.com*, an "Internet community for parents" founded by Elisa Ast All and Alvin All in 1996. The site is intended for consumers and presents accurate information. The best features of the site are the variety of choices and options that are presented for couples to consider for their birth, sample birth plans, rationales for having a birth plan, birthing stories, and a discussion board. There are no identifiable weaknesses. The text is available in Spanish, and the site is easy to understand and use.

Childbirth.org

http://www.childbirth.org

Childbirth.org is a comprehensive Web site that seeks to educate consumers about the birth process and their available options and to help ensure that they receive the best possible care. The philosophy of this organization is "birth is a natural process, not a medical procedure." The site is sponsored by Childbirth.org and clearly identifies additional monetary sponsors via advertisements on the main page. Robin Elise Weiss, a childbirth educator and doula, founded the site.

A wealth of information is presented on the site and includes topics such as episiotomies, fetal monitoring, cesarean section, newborn feeding, and vaginal birth after cesarean options. Information is also given on various leading childbirth methods (e.g., Lamaze, LeBoyer). The site features chat rooms, birth stories, and photos. Information is accurate and complete.

The most important strength of the site is the comprehensiveness of the information. However, some of the links that are provided are not functioning, although there are often several links given on any particular topic. Overall, the site is easy to use and is nicely organized, but the text is available only in English.

DadsWorld.com

http://www.dadsworld.com

DadsWorld.com is geared to expectant fathers. The purpose of the site is to provide information on fetal development and resources for new fathers. The site is produced by DadsWorld Enterprises, which publishes several magazines for fathers. An advisory board of health care professionals supervises information written for the site. Information is accurate and easy to understand. Highlighted features include attractive text and photos and departments related to pregnancy, babyhood, and toddlers. Sections on childbirth classes and questions for an expert are provided. There is also an opportunity for users to write articles for the site, review a checklist for pregnancy and postpartum, and browse the shopping area. The text is available only in English.

Evergreen Health Care Family Maternity Center

http://www.evergreenhealthcare.org/maternity/questions.asp

This site provides parents and potential parents with information on choosing an obstetric health care provider. Evergreen Health Care of Kirkland, Washington sponsors the site. Information provided on the site is current and accurate. The best features of the site include the different sections of questions to ask the potential provider, including qualifications, routine practices, and accessibility. Links to other sections that address high-risk pregnancy, special care nursery, family-friendly places (local only), and pondering parenthood are also given. Text, which is available only in English, is written at a low to average reading level. The site is easy to use and attractively designed.

The Interactive Pregnancy Calendar

http://www.parentsplace.com/pregnancy/calendar

This interactive Web site provides parents with a tool to build a day-by-day customized calendar detailing the development of a baby from before conception to birth. The site is sponsored by *Parents.com*, a part of the ivillage Network (a commercial "women's online network providing practical solutions and everyday support for women between the ages of 25 and 54"). The information, which is intended for consumers, is accurate. The best features include the month-by-month division of information, increasing the ease of information retrieval, detailed descriptions of developmental periods, and additional articles on topics relating to specific developmental periods. Excellent links are provided to *Parentsplace.com*. Users must register and activate a password to use this site. Even though registration is free, some individuals may view it as bothersome. Text is available only in English. Information is written at an average reading level, and the site is easy to use.

Pregnancy and Exercise

http://lifematters.com/medicalinfo.html

Pregnancy and Exercise provides extensive information geared to women who wish to maintain an exercise regime during pregnancy.

The site is sponsored by WorldWorks Unlimited and is intended for consumers. Factual information is presented on physiological changes associated with pregnancy that may change exercise abilities, general guidelines for exercise during pregnancy, effects of exercise that can affect pregnancy, and complications of pregnancy that may affect exercise ability, including contraindications. Mara V. Saulitis, MD, contributed the information for the site. The layout of the homepage is similar to the layout of a textbook page, which could be more interesting for the consumer. Information is provided only in English. The site is easy to use and presents information at a simple to medium reading level.

Pregnancy and HIV

http://www.hcfa.gov/hiv

The goal of the Health Care Financing Administration (HCFA) in sponsoring this Web site is to provide women and health care providers with information related to HIV infection and pregnancy. Information is current; the text is written at a low to average reading level. There are seven main categories to choose from on the homepage, which allows the user to focus on a topic of interest. The site includes a search engine and links to the main HCFA homepage. Text is in English only.

Pregnancy Bedrest

http://armstrong.son.wisc.edu/~son/bedrest

Pregnancy Bedrest is an information and support Web site for high-risk pregnant women on bedrest and their families. The site was developed by Judy Maloni, PhD, RN, FAAN, and includes a section for health care providers. Accurate and current information is provided at a low to average reading level. Important features of the site include stories, information for families, a support network, and a frequently asked questions page. No weak points are noted. Information is available only in English at this time.

The Teen Pregnancy and Parenting Place

http://www.hometown.aol.com/mnn1121

The Teen Pregnancy and Parenting Place is a support and resource network for pregnant and parenting teens. The sponsor of the site is not indicated; however, the information that is presented represents accurate and current information. The site is very comprehensive and focuses on positive and negative aspects of teen pregnancy and parenting. Other features include pen pals, chat rooms, a message board, and a stories section. No weaknesses are noted. The site provides information at a simple level that is appropriate for teens. It is easy to use and genuinely caters to teens. Information is written in English only.

Chapter 28

Prostate Cancer

Meredith Wallace, PhD, RN, CS-ANP

Prostate cancer is a malignancy that was once detected only in late stages, resulting in imminent death. More recently, the identification of the prostate-specific antigen has enabled health care providers to quickly and inexpensively diagnose and treat prostate cancer, resulting in both increased reports of the disease and increased survival. Prostate cancer is prevalent in older men. Presently, statistics show that the likelihood of developing prostate cancer increases from 1 in 2,667 for men ages 50 to 54 to 1 in 874 for men ages 55 to 59. The likelihood continues to increase to 1 in 346 for men ages 60 to 64, 1 in 174 for men ages 65 to 69, 1 in 115 for men ages 70 to 74, 1 in 90 for men ages 75 to 79, and 1 in 80 for men ages 80 to 84 (Litwin, 1994). Because of the increases in numbers and chronicity of men with this disease, there is a greater need for understandable information on diagnosis, treatment, and living with prostate cancer. The following Web sites are easily accessible.

American Cancer Society Prostate Cancer Resource Center

http://www3.cancer.org/cancerinfo
(Select "Prostate Cancer")

This site, part of the American Cancer Society's cancer resource center, gives general information on the disease, detection, risk factors, prevention, symptoms, and treatment options. Its purpose is to provide individuals with "answers to questions about the nature of cancer, its causes and risk factors." The site features an "Ask the Expert" bulletin board, where frequently asked questions about cancer are addressed by medical experts. Links to the "Man to Man" prostate cancer education and support program as well as to other Web sites are provided. The text is available in both English and Spanish.

The information is current and accurate. Users can sign up to receive e-mail updates on their particular type of cancer. Because all the links to prostate cancer information are on the left side of the main resource page, as opposed to within the main page, this is not the easiest site to navigate. Novice users may have trouble navigating. The main prostate cancer resource page gives only a brief description and links to other resources, but no specific information.

Cancernet

http://cancernet.nci.nih.gov/Cancer_Types/Prostate_Cancer.shtml

This Web site supplies facts on over 20 specific components of prostate cancer, ranging from an introduction to the disease to current research findings. The purpose of the site is to provide recent and accurate cancer information from the National Cancer Institute (NCI). The site is managed by the NCI's Office of Cancer Information, Communication, and Education. No credentials regarding the medical supervision of the site were provided.

The site provides an exhaustive amount of information on the disease and all related treatments, decisions, scientific information, and medical concerns. It also gives links to several other Web sites. The most important feature lies in the comprehensiveness of the information. This site is extraordinarily thorough in its coverage of the topic. However, its weakness lies within this strength. Because the site was intended for a wide target audience, from a consumer perspective, it contains too much information. By clicking the desired link or search function, for example, users are asked to select another link and may find themselves with a final product that is too difficult to understand or that is not what they were originally looking for. The text is in English only. Although the quality of the information is high, the vast amount of information and the difficulty navigating through it make the site consumer-unfriendly. This site is recommended only when the information needed supersedes what can be obtained from more user-friendly sites and then should be approached with assistance if available.

Cancer-Prostate.Com

http://www.cancer-prostate.com

As stated on the homepage, the purpose of this site is to provide free information on prostate cancer. The site was created by Faiyaaz Jhaveri, MD, a urologic oncologist and surgeon, fellowship-trained in prostate cancer from the Cleveland Clinic Foundation and practicing outside Orlando, FL. The site features a general introduction, definitions, treatment, and side effects. In addition, a bibliography is provided.

The site was created in 1999 and remains current and accurate. The definitions section provides clear explanations of the terminology related to the disease. The treatment section is clear and easy to understand. Side effects are listed by treatment and are presented in a relatively straightforward manner. Interestingly, the descriptions within each topic increase in complexity as the reader navigates through them. This is especially true in the treatment section, which provides a clear description of the treatment, followed by a "Cancer Control" section that would be beyond the comprehension level of the average consumer. At points the referencing of information and the high-level terminology may be too advanced for the average consumer. Although the author clearly is attempting to appeal to both consumers and clinicians, these complex explanations may be difficult and subsequently frustrating to read. Overall, the information on the site is accurate and would be a good source for both basic and more complex information about the disease. Text is written only in English.

Chapter 29

Sexually Transmitted Diseases

Carl A. Kirton, MA, RN, ANP-CS, ACRN and
Joseph P. Colagreco, MS, RN, ANP-CS

The following Web sites provide accurate and timely information on sexually transmitted diseases (STDs). For information on HIV/AIDS, see Chapter 20, which is devoted to the topic. Information alone can help prevent STDs, but once infected, individuals should use this information to seek appropriate treatment from a health care professional.

The Herpes Zone

http://www.herpeszone.com

This site is simple in structure, graphically pleasing, and "speaks" to a person with herpes. This is a good site for someone who is new to herpes and wants basic information. Examples of topic headings are "Living with Herpes," "Coping with Herpes," and "Herpes Management."

A disappointing feature of this site is under the link "Find Out How Others Are Coping with Herpes, Discover Support." In this link, there is only a small amount of useless text. The site could benefit from some interesting graphics—essentially there are none. The site has links to other sites that may be of interest, but at the time of this review several of the links were broken, and the ones that did work mostly led to pharmaceutical companies offering herpes drugs and other products. There is little here of interest to health care professionals.

I wannaknow.org: Answers to Your Questions About Teen Sexual Health and STD Prevention

http://www.iwannaknow.org

This site is sponsored by Merck and the American Social Health Association, a nonprofit organization dedicated to stopping STDs and their harmful consequences to individuals, families, and communities (*http://www.ashastd.org*). The site provides very basic information that is mostly in narrative form. There is a section on dealing with puberty, a FAQs site, and a chat room. There are two games that are meant to appeal to teens, but if you do not have macromedia shockwave as a browser plug-in, you are unable to play them.

This site attempts to appeal to the teen market. As an adult, however, I quickly lost interest.

Planned Parenthood

http://www.plannedparenthood.org

An organization with name recognition may be a popular site for patients to obtain information about their sexual health. This site is well designed and graphically pleasing to the eye. The information presented is up to date and accurate. For the most part, text is given in narrative form. In short, the site is adequate but would not be our preferred choice of sites for extensive information regarding STDs.

The Royal Adelaide Hospital Sexually Transmitted Disease Service

http://www.stdservices.on.net

This is the site for Clinic 275, which is located in Adelaide, South Australia. The clinic is part of the Royal Adelaide Hospital, founded in 1840 and incorporated under South Australia's Health Commission in October 1976. It is an accredited hospital. Clinic 275 offers free and confidential testing, along with diagnosis and treatment, of sexually transmitted infections (including HIV/AIDS). This is a site for individuals who suspect they have or simply want more information on an STD.

Pages are divided into the following topic areas: "Essential Facts," for men and women diagnosed with gonorrhea; "More Details," for students and clinicians; and "Diagnosis and Management Guidelines," for health care workers managing patients with gonorrhea. Also included are clinical photographs, statistics, annual and quarterly surveillance reports outlining the latest gonorrhea statistics in South Australia, and pamphlets that can be downloaded.

Patients will enjoy the audio pronunciation of medical terms (e.g., click on the word *gonorrhea* and hear an audio clip pronouncing it). Also impressive is the section "Having a Sexual Health Check-Up." It takes the reader through each step of the process, from reception and waiting, to consultation, to the examination and swab test, to blood tests and results, to treatment and follow-up. The text is accompanied by sharp graphics. Overall, it is rare for such a facility to have such an impressive Web site. It is highly recommended.

Thrive Online

http://thriveonline.oxygen.com

ThriveOnline was founded in 1996 as a joint venture between America Online and Time Inc. The site offers excellent information not only on STDs but also on a variety of other health-related topics.

With regard to STDs, a simple click on the "Sexuality" link brings the reader to a host of topics dealing with sex and sexuality. A simple search under "Reproductive Health" directs the reader to the STD section. STDs are listed with simple explanations and in some cases brilliant, clear photos to accompany some of the disorders.

The one drawback is that the ad banners that engulf the main content can be distracting.

Chapter 30

Sleep and Fatigue

Angela L. Hudson, PhD, RN and Kathryn A. Lee, PhD, RN, FAAN

This review highlights six Web sites related to sleep and fatigue that will be of interest to nurses and consumers. The following sites were among the top 20 "hits." The search words *fatigue* and *sleep*, using the search engine *yahoo.com*, yielded a total of 719 Internet sites related to these topics.

American Academy of Sleep Medicine

http://www.aasmnet.org

This is the official Web site of the American Academy of Sleep Medicine (AASM), a professional organization with members engaged in sleep disorders medicine and research. The goal of this site is to provide convenient access to sites related to sleep research, professional sleep organizations, and sleep medicine and practice guidelines. The majority of links are for professional purposes, such as the American Board of Sleep Medicine and the Medical School Education Committee. However, there is a link for consumers to take advantage of online purchase of patient education brochures. These "wellness booklets" are sold in lots of 50 for $35 for nonmembers of AASM. Examples of booklets include "Obstructive Sleep Apnea and Snoring" and "Sleep and Depression." "My Child Can't Sleep" and "My Child Snores" are examples of educational materials related to children and sleep. Because this site would not be a recommended first choice for lay consumers, it receives a "better than average" rating. For nurses, health educators, and other health care providers, this site receives an excellent rating, primarily for its inclusion of materials related to sleep problems in the pediatric population.

Fatigue: How to Know When to See a Doctor

http://www.cnn.com/health/9909/21/lack.of.energy

This Internet site, sponsored by the Cable News Network (CNN), was written by a physician associated with *WebMd.com* (a large commercial Web site for health professionals). The site describes the etiology of fatigue and helps consumers decide when to see a health care provider. It gives a description of fatigue related to lifestyle (new motherhood, stress, alcohol use, or caffeine intake) and medical conditions (diabetes, anemia, and hypothyroidism). The site's intended audience is consumers.

The best feature of this site is its links to health-related news stories regarding women, men, diet/fitness, and children. There is also a link to the National Sleep Foundation Web site (see separate entry), a chronic fatigue syndrome site, and *WebMd.com*. Text is clear and easy to read. A major drawback, however, is that the site appears not to be updated regularly. Also, with no e-mail contact address provided, there is no way to submit questions. The text is in English, but other sites, related to news-breaking CNN reports, are referenced in Spanish, Italian, Portuguese, and Danish. This site receives an average rating for quality and level of information.

Fibromyalgia

http://www.nursece.com/onlinecourses/908.html

This is a Web site for continuing education on fibromyalgia, a chronic illness in which fatigue and nonrestorative sleep are characteristic symptoms. The site sponsor is the National Center of Continuing Education (a commercial provider of continuing education courses for nurses). This text-based, noninteractive site allows nurses to complete a continuing education program on fibromyalgia. The information, however, is very useful for consumers. The goal of the site is to describe the prevalence, etiology, and management strategies for FM. Although the intended audience is nurses, the site can also be helpful for recently diagnosed patients. Information is available only in English. Patient education and management strategies for such self-care behaviors as sleep hygiene, exercise, and cognitive-behavioral approaches are informative. A case study, in accordance with nursing practice guidelines, is also provided.

The information is accurate, comprehensive, and objective. However, no date is given for future postings of new information or research findings. Although this site lacks all graphic elements, the text-based design makes it easy and fast to download information. There are no links to other sleep or fatigue Web sites. This site receives an average rating.

National Sleep Foundation

http://www.sleepfoundation.org

The homepage for the National Sleep Foundation (NSF) provides information on particular sleep disorders, current sleep research, and funding opportunities. Topics covered include a definition of the nature of sleep, the impact of poor sleep and fatigue on health and productivity, and sleep strategies for shift workers. There is also a separate and distinct category of information on issues surrounding women and sleep. A sleep diary can be downloaded for self-care assessment and management of insomnia.

This Web site is well designed, colorful, comprehensive, and easily hyperlinked to sleep-related issues and affiliated organizations. There is also an e-mail address for sleep inquiries (*nsf@sleepfoundation.org*). The site does not include product advertising. It has a consumer-oriented sleep survey. Anonymity in participating in the survey entails downloading the survey and mailing it to NSF after completion.

Overall, this site is excellent for both nurses and consumers.

National Women's Health Information Center

http://www.4women.gov

The Office of Research on Women's Health, Department of Health and Human Services at the National Institutes of Health, sponsors this Web site. Its purpose is to serve as a gateway for consumers to link to sites, read, or download information pertaining to women's health issues. This is a hyperlinked site, allowing independent searching. For example, entering the word *sleep* or *fatigue* will link the user to research papers, statistics, and related organizations.

The site is updated almost daily. Users can call a toll-free number (800-994-9622) to reach a referral specialist, who can clarify information and identify appropriate federal and private-sector health resources. The site is user-friendly and graphically appealing. The extent and quality of information provided are excellent.

Restless Legs Syndrome Foundation

http://www.rls.org

Sleep is often difficult to initiate for those who suffer from restless legs syndrome (RLS). Consequently, fatigue is a common complaint. The RLS Foundation Web site is a good source for information on this condition. Users can participate in online support groups and learn of the latest research findings, as well as regional programs and opportunities for research funding. The site is user-friendly and graphically appealing. Overall, it merits a very good rating for both consumers and nurses who work with populations of at-risk groups, such as those with chronic iron-deficiency anemia.

--- **Chapter 31**

Smoking Cessation

Meg Smirnoff, MPH, RN, FNP

The stages of readiness to stop smoking range from "not ready to think about it" (precontemplative), to "thinking about it" (contemplative), to "ready to commit and to act" (the action stage), then maintenance of the healthful action. Studies have shown that 80% of smokers are in the precontemplative stage, at which point a health professional will have little success as a change agent. The sites reviewed here may help encourage those who are thinking about quitting to become more active in breaking the habit.

About.com: Smoking Cessation

http://quitsmoking.about.com

This is a highly interactive and stylized site that attempts to present all topics related to quitting smoking. The site "explores the total quit smoking experience" and has titles on traditional, nontraditional and wacky treatments. Topics include cigars, pregnancy, teen smoking, women's health, updates on the tobacco industry lawsuit settlement, and tobacco advertisers.

About.com is a privately held company. The site is geared toward consumers, with commercial tie-ins to markets that may interest them. The information is current and accurate.

One of the best features of the site is the link to the "No Smoking Cafe" (*clever.net/chrisco/nosmoke/stop.html?*), which is hosted by the guide of *quitsmoking.com* and is more personal, emotive, and "schmaltzy" than more objectively written sites. The site is fun, lively, and easy to use.

Quit4life

http://www.quit4life.com

This Web site, directed at teenagers, melds emotionally charged stories of four young people with their smoking cessation issues in a factually correct yet still "cool" manner. The site is sponsored by Health Canada. The information is current and accurate.

The site does not "force" the message; rather, the storylines flow in such a way that the reader controls the amount of hard data to see. He or she may choose to follow just the dramatic story line or to view any or all of the information. The site is available in English and French. The language is simple; much of it is in "teen speak." It is visually attractive and engrossing, with fun graphics.

Quitnet

http://www.quitnet.org

This is a highly informative, inclusive site that offers the best of the quitting guides from almost all available resources. The site includes a broad range of information and yet is easily personalized to the needs of each respondent (e.g., "My Quit Calendar," "My Quit Date," and an anniversary e-mail sent for long-term support). It is one of several sites of "Join Together," a substance abuse online resource based at the Boston University School of Public Health. The site is intended for consumers, yet is broad and substantive enough to satisfy professionals. Information is current and accurate.

The site has many selections, including peer support groups, quitting guides, referrals to local programs, quitting-aid product reviews, and tobacco-related news stories. Of note, the site also addresses the needs of those who use smokeless tobacco. The text is in English only. The level of information ranges from average to high. The site is easy to navigate and graphically appealing.

Soyouwanna.com

http://soyouwanna.com/site/syws/quit/quit.html

This is an engaging presentation of quit options and appropriate referrals that relates as a partner in the struggle with the smoker rather
than as a dryly scientific authority. The site is written in a playful,
conspiratorial voice as one of a series of exploratory services whose
self-described purpose is "life explained." Soyouwanna.com (SYW) is
a privately held company backed by Inculab Inc. Its mission is to be
a "provider of explanatory lifestyle content."

The site is directed at consumers, with strong vendor tie-ins. Information is current and accurate. The site has information on available
chemical and natural treatments, reviews books, has a member bulletin
board, and links to related SYW sites, such as "White Teeth," "Lower
Cholesterol," and "Help a Friend with a Drug Problem." The text is
available only in English. The level of information is average. The site
is fun and entertaining.

_____ Chapter 32

Spinal Cord Injury

Jill M. Goldstein, MA, RN, MS

These sites are designed for the beginner through advanced internet surfer. The detail you will find will provide the patient, family, or day-to-day surfer simply interpreted information on what a spinal cord injury is, demographics related to such, how it affects daily living, recommended spinal cord rehab centers, current Web links for current research studies, and more.

Cure Paralysis Now

http://www.cureparalysis.org

This site is dedicated to all who are involved with or affected by spinal cord injury, especially researchers and clinicians in multidisciplinary fields of study that may relate to the advancement of the healing, or cure of spinal cord paralysis. It is sponsored by the actor Christopher Reeve. Information is at a moderate to advanced level and is current and accurate. The site is easy to navigate.

Eastern Paralyzed Veterans Association

http://www.epva.org

The Eastern Paralyzed Veterans Association (EPVA) is dedicated to enhancing the lives of veterans with a spinal cord injury or disease by assuring quality health care, promoting research, and advocating for civil rights and independence. EPVA is a chapter of the congressionally chartered Paralyzed Veterans of America and has over 2,000 members residing in New York, New Jersey, Pennsylvania, and Connecticut.

EPVA is a not-for-profit organization based in Jackson Heights, New York. It maintains offices in Buffalo and New York, New York; Newark, New Jersey; and Philadelphia, Pennsylvania.

Since its founding in 1946, EPVA has enabled members, as well as other persons with disabilities, to lead full and productive lives. All of its services, from benefits counseling to wheelchair sports, are supported through greeting-card solicitations and other fund-raising programs.

An important feature is that one can request free written materials from the site. Information is also available in Spanish. The level of information is simple, and the site is easy to navigate.

National Spinal Cord Injury Association

http://www.spinalcord.org

In order to assist the 7,800 individuals who sustain a SCI each year, and the 400,000 persons living with spinal cord injuries, the National Spinal Cord Injury Association (NSCIA) was established in 1948. The NSCIA has many chapters throughout the United States. Some members have physical disabilities while others do not. Chapter members participate in a variety of activities. They work with local and national officials and agencies to develop better programs and services and act as community advocates for improved access, housing, transportation, employment, and leisure time activities for disabled people. Peer support and other services are also provided. These are fundamental aspects of living that 500,000 people with spinal cord injuries or diseases must cope with after they have been rehabilitated and have returned to community life. More and more persons are getting involved in activities of the NSCIA. Through the collective efforts of staff, chapters, board members, and other volunteers, the Association is improving care, producing results in research, and addressing everyday living issues that confront all people who use wheelchairs.

Information is current and accurate. Important features are the description of regional systems of care and support, research, and resolution of problems and issues. Wording is simple and the site is easy to navigate. Information is in English only.

Spinal Cord Injury—For Your Information

http://www.tbi-sci.org/scifyi

The SCI-FYI is a comprehensive resource guide intended for anyone in Santa Clara Valley (and beyond) needing information on services related to spinal cord injury—from the rehab professional looking for services to help a client, to family members searching for programs to assist their loved one, to the individual with a spinal cord injury who wants to improve his or her personal situation. As with any directory of community agencies, it will need updating by the time it is posted, but the majority of information should remain current and valuable for those seeking resources. The site is easy to use, and colorful. Information is in English only.

Spinal Cord Injury Information Network

http://www.spinalcord.uab.edu

The Medical Rehabilitation Research and Training Center on Secondary Conditions of Spinal Cord Injury at University Alabama at Birmingham-Spain Rehabilitation Center has a series of 18 information sheets on selected topics related to spinal cord injury (SCI). These concise four to six page information sheets are written at different knowledge levels and for different audiences and include additional print and audiovisual resources. The intended audience is individuals with spinal cord injury, family/friends, and rehabilitation clinical team members. The information is current and accurate. Wording is simple, and the site is easy to navigate. The site is also available in Spanish.

Spinal Cord Injury Ring

http://www.tbi-sci.org/sciring

The SCI Ring is a collection of web sites that share a common interest in spinal cord injury. All members of the ring have a graphic logo and a link to other ring members. Its goal is to include pages that include resources, news, research, and experiences regarding spinal cord injury. Professionals, organizations, and individuals are invited to join.

The site is owned by The TBI & SCI Projects, Santa Clara Valley Medical Center. Information is current and accurate. An important feature is the ability to start your own chat rooms—a lot of individual needs can be chased down here. Language is in layman's terms, and the site is easy to navigate. Information is in English only.

Chapter 33

Stroke

Betty J. Furr, MSN, RN, CRRN

S troke is one of the leading causes of death and disability in the United States. It affects a large percentage of the population directly, as stroke survivors, or indirectly, as family members or loved ones of stroke survivors.

The chronic, sometimes debilitating nature of this disorder often motivates stroke survivors and their families to look for answers. In this information age of computer technology, it is natural to search the Internet. The knowledge found can enhance self-care, but it is important for consumers to recognize that all information or advice available on the Internet may not be suitable.

Many universities and health care organizations have Web sites that provide the needed information. However, some sites are produced or sponsored by individuals or groups with limited qualifications to offer advice. The sites evaluated here can be safely recommended to stroke survivors and their families as reputable, current, and accurate.

American Stroke Association

http://www.strokeassociation.org

This site is sponsored by the American Stroke Association (ASA), a division of the American Heart Association. It is an extensive repository of information on stroke and related disorders and is appropriate for both consumers and professionals.

The "Heart and Stroke A–Z Guide" allows consumers to educate themselves on the latest information on stroke prevention, treatment and services. Professionals can find information on research grants, scientific papers, conferences, and services.

The link to the ASA site from the homepage of the American Heart Association (AHA) (*www.americanheart.org*) is very confusing. The AHA site is crammed with drop-down menus, multiple frames, and competing color schemes. The link to ASA is through "atrial fibrillation." It would be clearer and more direct to list "stroke" or "cerebral vascular accident" as the link. For this reason, it is best to access the ASA site directly. For a review of AHA site, see Chapter 19.

All of the information can be easily understood by most consumers. The site is simply designed and easy to navigate. Text is in English only.

National Institute of Neurological Disorders and Stroke

http://www.ninds.nih.gov

The National Institute of Neurological Disorders and Stroke, part of the National Institute of Health, is the leading supporter of research on the causes, prevention, diagnosis, and treatment of neurological disorders. Its Web site targets professionals; however, there are links to consumer-specific sites. Information is current and reliable, although the level may be too high for the average consumer. The best feature is the *ClinicalTrials.gov* link for medical research (developed by the National Library of Medicine). It lists trials currently recruiting select consumer participants.

The site has minimal frames and drop-down menus. This contributes to the ease of use because the site offers few distractions.

National Stroke Association

http://www.stroke.org

This site, sponsored by the National Stroke Association (NSA), offers comprehensive information on stroke prevention, treatment, rehabilitation, research, and support for stroke survivors and their families. The information is also useful for the general public and health care professionals.

As a resource for physicians, nurses, and other health care professionals, the NSA publishes the latest research findings and clinical updates as a component of its continuing education programs.

The site is easy to navigate using simple point-and-click options. This is helpful for stroke survivors. The text is in English only. Overall, the site is well organized and graphically appealing.

Chapter 34

Travel Considerations

Felissa R. Lashley, PhD, RN, ACRN, FAAN

There are many health factors to consider when traveling to another country. Are vaccinations required to obtain a visa? Is the water safe to drink? Are there any contagious disease outbreaks occurring? The travel health sites reviewed here provide helpful information for travelers, much of it specific to particular destinations.

International Travel and Health: Vaccination Requirements and Health Advice (World Health Organization)

http://www.who.int/ith

This site emphasizes vaccination requirements, major diseases related to international travel, and geographic distribution of health hazards and risks related to the environment, as well as food and drink safeguards and sexual transmission rates. It is produced by the World Health Organization for consumers and health professionals. Information is current and accurate.

In addition to information on vaccinations, the site has information on special situations, such as extended travel, pregnancy, chronic illness, blood transfusion, malaria, and emergency treatment. A weak point is that it does not have extensive disease-by-disease information or extensive country-by-country information. Text is available in English and French. The site is easy to use.

International Travel Medicine Clinic

http://www.hsc.unt.edu/patientcare/itmc/travel.htm

This site has information for those making travel plans, including general precautions, such as for food and beverage safeguards and vaccine information, as well as specific disease information. The site is produced by the University of North Texas Health Science Center at Fort Worth. It is intended for consumers but is helpful for health professionals. Information is current and accurate.

The best features of the site are its tips on pretravel planning, specific information on malaria prevention, and health hazard information by destination.

The site is a little difficult to navigate. There is limited information at the first level, which gives descriptions of hazards by country. Users have to click again on a particular disease to get full information. Information is in English only.

The site is straightforward and simply designed. Pages do not pop up directly. Users must first pass through the main homepage, search, then "sign" a user's agreement.

Travel Health Online

http://www.tripprep.com

This site provides health information for travelers on specific illnesses, from altitude sickness to yellow fever, as well as information related to specific destinations. It is produced by Shoreland Inc., a company that publishes information from publicly available sources, mostly government entities, from around the world. The publisher does not investigate the accuracy or completeness of the content references on the site. The site is intended for the general public. Information seems accurate. Features include destination information, information on specific health conditions related to travel, and names and addresses of travel medicine providers in the United States and worldwide. The site requires Microsoft or Netscape Browser 4.0 or later. It is attractive and easy to use.

Travel Medicine Program, Health Canada

http://www.hc-sc.gc.ca/hpb/lcdc/osh/mp_e.html

This site provides health information, recommendations, and advice for travelers. It is produced by the Population and Public Health Branch of Health Canada, an organization that provides national leadership to develop health policy and promote disease prevention and healthy living for all Canadians. Persons planning international travel and health professionals providing counsel to them are the intended audience. Information is current and accurate.

The site covers current disease outbreak information, immunization recommendations for international travel, general health advice for international travelers, and specific prevention and treatment guidelines. There is also travel advice by country.

One weak point is the lack of an alphabetical listing of diseases. Text is in English and French. The site is easy to use.

Travelers' Health (CDC)

http://www.cdc.gov/travel

This site provides health-related recommendations for specific countries as well as information on specific diseases and health issues. It is produced by the National Center for Infectious Diseases of the Centers for Disease Control and Prevention. Consumers and health professionals are the intended audience. Information is current and accurate.

There are sections on destinations, specific diseases, with an emphasis on travelers' health, specific disease outbreak information, tips on food and water safety, insect protection, information on vaccinations and where to get them, and specific information for cruise ship passengers and airline travelers. Sections on traveling with children and for travelers with special needs, including immune suppression, are available. Links to a number of related sites, such as the World Health Organization (see separate entry), are provided. There is also an "In the News" feature. Text is in English, with some specific information in Spanish and Portuguese. The site is attractive and easy to use.

Chapter 35

Women's Health

Diana L. Taylor, PhD, RN and Gina M. Wade, MS, RN

U sing multiple Web search engines as well as our own knowledge of women's health-related Web sites, we reviewed approximately 40 commercial, government, and organization sites. We chose these sites on the following merits: current information, accuracy, completeness, and bias. We looked for credible authors (identified credentials), dated and cited sources, and funding sources. We also looked at the level of interactivity and community available on the site. A credentialed professional with experience in the condition discussed should always monitor the community. Interactivity provides individualized information for a consumer that is more useful and empowering.

We excluded a number of popular Web sites that have been developed for primarily entertainment purposes, such as WebMD, Thrive Online, and iVillage, as we found it difficult to differentiate between content that included current, complete, and accurate information and entertainment content. The information provided can be misleading and biased and is usually based on the amount of funding provided by pharmaceutical or device manufacturing companies. Many of the discussion boards and communities are not managed by health professionals and can lead to misinformation and increased confusion.

In addition to evaluating women's health Web sites for currency, accuracy, and completeness, we selected sites based on evidence of bias or statement of philosophy. All but one of the sites we chose clearly states its philosophy of women's health (*http://www.womens healthnetwork.org*), and only two sites provide information clearly focused on issues of gender and cultural diversity (*http://www. 4women.gov*; and *http://www.womenshealthnetwork.org*).

Women's health information on the Net appears dominated by a biomedical approach—focused on biologically treatable and definable issues. Although focused on diseases specific to women, a biomedical approach isolates health and illness as biological variables distinct from a wider social context and has its limits to improving individual health and wellness. Diagnosis and treatment that are entirely biologically based do not address the broader health concerns of women, who tend to describe their health status in subjective, contextual ways. Although medical professionals have been dedicated to quality health care, women's health is more than disease and biological conditions. Gender, culture, social relationships, and political-economic factors influence a woman's ability to access health information and use the information for personal health care decision making. Superior health information resources must address the broader health concerns of women beyond biological dimensions of disease.

We must remember that all information, whether written, oral, or electronic, reflects cultural norms in the health information they supply, or fail to supply.

Some questions that may help to evaluate Web site content for legitimacy, accuracy, and bias are as follows: Is the health-related information written from a woman's perspective? Is the information culturally appropriate, or are cultural/ethnic differences among women described? Is the information provided so women can participate actively and knowledgeably in decisions concerning their bodies and health?

In the following review, you will find three organizational Web sites, two commercial sites, and one government site for women and health care professionals. All but one is specifically focused on women's health and represents a global health Web site with high-level health information on a range of women's health issues (*http://www.health watch.medscape.com*). Two sites were chosen for their emphasis on women's health research or health information analysis and policy (*http://www.womens-health.org* and *http://www.womenshealthnet work.org*). One commercial site (*http://www.womens-health.com*), a government Web site (*http:www.4women.gov*), and a nonprofit organization site (*http://www.healthywomen.org*) provide high-quality, interactive information on a wide range of medical and health issues important to women.

CBS Healthwatch by Medscape

http://www.healthwatch.medscape.com

This is a general consumer health information site with health channels, including women's health. It is a free membership site that provides "high-quality information and interactive tools to help consumers and their families manage their daily personal health." CBS is the producer of the site, along with pharmaceutical companies sponsoring different segments of the site. It is for consumers. Membership is also offered for health professionals at *Medscape.com*, a large medical Web site.

Content is written by an editorial staff and is reviewed by physicians (no nurses). The sources are cited and dated. The articles are categorized by date and on the basis of the reader's level of health literacy—basic, advanced, and professional. All articles are listed by most current date. Although the women's health channel has only a few of the larger major illness conditions specific to women (i.e., osteoporosis, PMS, breast cancer, STDs), it appears to be developing more. By using the health topics form A–Z, you can find any other information. Topics that are fully developed feature news updates, discussion boards, and interactive tools. A professional nurse moderates the discussion boards.

Important features of the site are as follows:

- Health Channels—libraries of information with different levels of literacy and interactive tools to track health goals
- Health Manager—includes a health calendar for logging meals, etc.
- Health Mates—community discussion board, which is moderated by a professional
- Drug Directory—list of community organizations involved in particular health conditions.

The site also has access to Medline and a medical test handbook.

Weak points are that it has a medical rather than a health or wellness focus. Also, the site does not modify the information for ethnicity, such as nutrition information specific for Latina, African American, or Asian women. Another drawback is that users must complete a profile before using any interactive tools. This information is probably used for marketing and research purposes. Because certain pharmaceutical companies sponsor a considerable portion of the educational information, certain biases cannot be ruled out.

Text is in English only. The site is fairly easy to use, with clear, concise information presented in a logical order. It is not cluttered or distracting.

National Women's Health Information Center

http://www.4women.org

or

http://www.4women.gov

The National Women's Health Information Center (NWHIC), a service of the Office on Women's Health of the Department of Health and Human Services, provides women's health-related material developed by the Department of Health and Human Services, the Department of Defense, other federal agencies, and private-sector resources. Resources for NWHIC are selected primarily from U.S. government agencies; national voluntary, nonprofit, and professional organizations serving the public interest; universities, other educational institutions, and libraries; state and local government agencies offering information services beyond their geographic boundaries; and organizations partnering with government agencies to provide information to the public.

There are a few for-profit organizations that are included in this site. They provide free health information. They do not promote the sale of the products or lobbying efforts. These materials include online journals and news Web sites. Large indexes of health and human services information are provided free of charge as a public service by a commercial entity.

Consumers and health care providers are the intended audience. The site presents a detailed program regarding pregnancy, violence against women, and heart disease. It is very interactive and informative on every aspect. The FAQ section has lots of helpful information on a wide range of topics, with sources cited and dates given. Most of the health content is found by the "search" function on the site. This is one of the few sites that includes focuses on women with disabilities and minority women, with photos of Latina, black, and older women.

Important features of the site include links to other government-sponsored women's health sites, such as the Food and Drug Administration's Office of Women's Health and the National Institutes of

Health's Office of Research on Women's Health, and a calendar of upcoming events for consumers and professionals.

This is an especially good resource for women with disabilities, covering disease information and laws and regulations related to access to care. An 800 number is provided for additional information.

The site gives daily news updates on women's health legislation and related issues. In the "Health Professional" section there is a vast array of information (e.g., clinical trials for patients, online Merck Manual, publications, pictures and diagrams). The "Body Image" section covers prevention and health promotion strategies (i.e., exercise/nutrition). It has links to many other sites. The "Guest Editor" section features health experts who write on particular topics. It is very informative, with easy access to a wide range of topics from specific experts.

One weak point is the functionality of quizzes. "Error" appeared when attempting to take the quizzes using both Internet Explorer and Netscape browsers. When requesting more information on a particular subject, the site returns to the main page, which is confusing.

The site is easy to navigate and graphically appealing. There is a lot of information in Spanish. However, because it has so many links, users can become confused.

National Women's Health Network

http://www.womenshealthnetwork.org

This is the homepage of the National Women's Health Network, the first nonprofit health advocacy organization (founded in 1975) to successfully influence federal health policy. The site gives information about the organization's advocacy efforts (breast cancer, menopause, osteoporosis, hormone replacement therapy, health care and welfare reform, HIV/AIDS and women, safe drugs and devices, and reproductive health) and offers the extensive Health Information Clearinghouse, which analyzes information and resources from science and industry to assist consumers in making better health care decisions. The purpose of the site is to inform the public of policy issues regarding women's health and to provide well-researched information on a variety of women's health issues.

The National Women's Health Network is supported by 10,000 individual and 300 organizational members. The network does not accept funding from pharmaceutical companies or medical device manufacturers. The site is for consumers and health professionals interested in policy analysis and woman-focused, research-based critique of women's health issues.

This is one of the few sites that states a refreshingly clear philosophy that is focused on health and illness within a social, political, and environmental context. Health information on the site is minimal. However, comprehensive packets of information can be ordered online. There is a descriptions of how the site's information is compiled (by use of interns, with expert review and fact checking).

Important features of the site include the following:

- This is the only source for policy analysis of important women's health issues.
- Health information extends beyond the usual biomedical perspective and raises questions about selected treatments or existing knowledge (e.g., breast cancer detection methods, hormone therapy, drug safety, and reproductive rights).
- Health information packets focus on helping women make educated health care decisions and include selected articles, a glossary, and an extensive annotated bibliography on a wide range of women's health issues not included in other Web sites (e.g., AIDS in women, chronic fatigue syndrome, lesbian health, breast implants, bias against women in medicine, and abortion).
- Fact sheets can be purchased online (e.g., breast cancer in minority women, tamoxifen use for healthy women, Raloxifene, breast biopsies and breast cancer surgery, and microbicides for the prevention of sexually transmitted diseases).
- "Taking Hormones and Women's Health" is the only publication with a balanced, research-based perspective and includes an excellent section on decision making for hormone use.
- The site focuses on cultural differences among women and their health disparities.

A weak point is that there is limited online information for consumers, although Web site expansion is in progress. The site has a simple format and is easy to use.

National Women's Health Resource Center

http://www.healthywomen.org

The National Women's Health Resource Center (NWHRC) is a nonprofit organization dedicated to educating consumers about women's health and wellness. Services include providing numerous publications on a variety of women's health topics for a fee and sponsoring a database of national, regional, and local health resources without cost. It is a forum for presenting relatively unbiased women's health information. As the national clearinghouse for women's health information, the goal of NWHRC is to provide access to women's health information and resources from a broad range of sources. According to the producers of the site, the information offered is comprehensive, objective, and supported by an advisory council comprised of the nation's leading medical and health experts. One problem is that members of the advisory board are not listed. Also, the content is not cited or dated.

The NWHRC receives educational grants sponsored by consumer products manufacturers and the pharmaceutical industry, such as Procter and Gamble, Johnson & Johnson, Eli Lilly, Parke Davis, and Healthy Woman. The producers of the site discuss working with leading health experts and organizations in women's health, but they do not provide biographies or any information on these experts. The intended audience is consumers.

Some topics are not yet developed; however there are many developed, diversified subjects with information on conferences, organizations, and resources relating to each health topic. The content is organized according to a diagnostic model: overview, diagnosis, treatment, and so on. Source and date of information are not provided. Names of other health Web sites, with descriptions of content, however, are given. Access to multimedia resources is furnished in many health areas. Pamphlets, videos, books, and other resources can be ordered online.

Users can answer surveys designed to update the producers on consumers' interests and knowledge base. The site presents up-to-date news on women's health via the Reuter's news service.

Important features of the site include:

- Point of View—Different opinions from experts referring to questions asked by consumers. This information appears nonbiased, objective, comprehensive, and well organized.
- A–Z Health Center—contains not only explanations of condition but also prevention and a list of questions to ask providers during visits
- Updated News—covers specific women's health conditions, current events, and conferences
- Library—features multimedia content, publications, and books

- Health Services—provides names of organizations and clinics in a particular geographical area

Weak points include the following: Questions are not answered by health care providers on the discussion board but by people who have logged on to the site. The board seems inactive and unmonitored. The content is all text, no graphics or photos. Information may be too sophisticated for average consumers. The content is not cited or dated.

The site is easy to use and navigate. There are no more than two screen scrolls for each page. The content is to the point, clear, and concise without being vague or misleading.

Society for Women's Health Research

http://www.womens-health.org

The Society for Women's Health Research is a nonprofit organization founded in 1990 to advocate for increased research funding for women's health as well as for the participation of women in clinical trials. The organization's Web site offers research-based information and referral sources on gender-specific conditions to consumers, health care professionals, and researchers. Although its perspective emphasizes a biomedical disease focus, this is one of the few sites that provides research-based knowledge on women's health conditions and gender-based biology.

The site has a host of sponsors, including pharmaceutical companies, that do not appear to influence the content. The health information is limited at the site and relies on linking consumers to outside sources. Information is referenced and dated.

Important features include:

- Women's health facts and links, which provide research-based facts and lists organizations that are involved with the general women's health field and specific diseases and conditions (e.g., breast cancer, cardiovascular diseases, and mental health)
- A compilation of Internet myths about women's health (e.g., tampons and asbestos, tumor marker for ovarian cancer)
- An extensive additional links section to government, private, and nonprofit sites related to women's health
- A compilation of grants available in women's health research and sex-based biology, as well as information about clinical trial participation

Weak points of the site are that it is limited to a biomedical and disease-specific perspective that is not clearly stated. Also, the purpose of the site is not easily understood, because it focuses only on gender without consideration of cultural and ethnic differences within gender. Public education materials are limited, and a review of information under the topic "Premenstrual Dysphoric Disorder" had some inaccuracies and was biased to pharmacological treatment.

Overall, the site is well organized, uncluttered, and easy to use. There are no sponsor advertisements.

Women's Health Interactive

http://www.womens-health.com

This site comprises multidisciplinary health education resources that are accessible to consumers and health care professionals. The purpose of the site is consumer education and it provides advertising space for advertisers aiming to communicate their services to women.

The site's management team is made up of physicians and nurses. Women's Health Interactive has several affiliates—the National Headache Foundation, the National Council on Women's Health, and Women's Work Inc.—and one sponsor, Glaxo Wellcome Inc., which has provided an unrestricted grant for the headache center.

Information, which appears complete and unbiased, covers a wide range of women's health concerns. However, it does not cover family health or other conditions and problems. The structure of the content is well thought out and designed and follows typical learning theories (i.e., assess, learn, interact, action plan). The content is not cited or dated, but there is a copyright date. The site is very interactive and uses surveys for information gathering regarding consumers' knowledge base. Some links are outdated.

Important features of the site include the following:

- Personal Assessment—consumers can assess their knowledge of a certain topic
- Health Centers—cover gynecology, headache, heart, mental health, infertility, midlife, natural health, nutrition, and personal development
- Research Center—presents completed research and upcoming research in selected areas
- Personal Stories—contains frequently asked questions

- Community Center—incorporates discussion boards on topics such as heart disease, infertility, menopause, mental health, journaling, and women's media

Although the "Community Center" section is well organized and moderated by professionals, there is very little activity in the few "communities" that are available. Although information on specific health conditions was factual and up to date, it was very basic, with no links given to additional information.

The site is organized, uncluttered, and easy to navigate, and there are sponsor advertisements. Text is in English, although some information in the "Gynecological Health Center" section is in German.

Chapter **36**

Wound and Ostomy Care

Dorothy C. Visco, BSN, RN, CWCN and
Susan J. Wren, BSN, RN, CWCN, COCN

T his chapter provides information on serious and chronic wounds, such as pressure sores and ostomies. Readers will find practical information on treatment, maintenance, and various products.

WOUND CARE

Skinwound.com

http://www.skinwound.com

The purpose of the site is to provide health care professionals and consumers with the latest information and resources on wound care essentials. It is the property of CompAssure Inc., which is the exclusive online distributor of Hyperion Medical wound care products.

The homepage directs you to three major areas of interest. The first section reviews wound dressing products in seven different categories: wound cleansers, hydrogels, hydrocolloids, alginates, gauze dressings, skin protectants, and tapeless bandages. The second section, "The Online Training Manual," is the main feature of this site. The manual is laid out in textbook fashion with a detailed outline at the beginning.

It covers nutrition and wound healing, risk assessment, documentation, and wound assessment. The wound assessment section reviews the etiology of pressure and vascular ulcers and gives photos as examples. The third section provides nursing care plans and case studies, focusing on the treatment of pressure ulcers, vascular ulcers, and burns. The plans and case studies, however, focus on the company's specific products instead of generic categories of products.

The site does not have links to related sites. Information is in English only.

Wound Care Information Network

http://www.medicaledu.com/wndguide.htm

This site is maintained by Cyber Group Development Inc. It is intended for health care professionals. However, it can serve as a valuable tool for consumers interested in obtaining detailed information on wound care.

The homepage is divided into four levels and "Hot Topics," which include a "search" feature of the site, weekly e-mail updates on wound care news, and a global wound care discussion forum. The discussion forum allows consumers to monitor conversations or to ask questions of the forum group regarding wound-related issues.

Level 1 covers the etiology of different types of chronic wounds, including pressure, arterial, venous, and diabetic. Information is given on wound documentation, pressure ulcer staging, and wound healing. Level 2 addresses the topics of wound infection versus contamination, burns, treatment modalities, and the various methods of wound debridement. Level 3 reviews topical wound dressings and gives a manufacturer's index for wound products. In addition, there is a review of tissue engineering as well as Medicare coverage criteria for support surfaces and wound dressings. Level 4 is geared to the nursing/medical professional and addresses legal and documentation issues as well as information on support groups for patients and practitioners.

Individuals with no exposure to medical terminology may have difficulty understanding some of the site content. Links to related sites are not provided. Text is in English only.

The site is easy to navigate. Many of the content areas include color photos to enhance the text.

OSTOMY CARE

Convatec Connection: Your Online Connection to Quality Information on Ostomy, Wound, and Skin Care

http://www.convatec.com

This site is produced by Convatec, a manufacturer of ostomy, wound, and skin care products. Convatec is part of the Bristol-Myers Squibb Co. The site gives product and company information, lists support groups and provides reimbursement information for customers. A separate version of the site is available for health care professionals. The intended audience is customers with ostomies and medical professionals.

An extensive dictionary of medical terms related to ostomy is given. The site also offers product training, with written instructions and pictures for visual demonstration. A free product sample can be sent to customers on request. A helpful "Hospital to Home" section explains surgical procedures and gives recommendations for the most common difficulties that can be encountered at home.

Users must download Real Player to view product videos (available free at a separate Web site).

Ostomy education booklets are available in English and Spanish. Other languages available are German, French, and Italian. The site is well organized and easy to use.

Hollister Inc.

http://www.hollister.com

The purpose of this site is to inform users of Hollister products, and to assist customers in finding ostomy products that meet their needs. The site is produced by Hollister Inc., a leader in health care product manufacturing for more than 77 years. Hollister has a worldwide presence in 91 countries. The site's intended audience is health care professionals and patients with ostomies. Information is current and accurate.

The site lists other sites/organizations that can provide additional information for patients with certain diseases. A questionnaire is available to assist in determining the best ostomy product for patients with pouching problems. Questions can be submitted to an enterostomal therapy nurse for additional assistance. Users can order free samples before making a purchase. Ostomy education booklets are available in English, Portuguese, and Spanish.

Adobe Acrobat is needed for viewing the "Hollister Ostomy Product Reference Guide," but free installation of the Acrobat reader is provided on the site.

Explanations are given in simple terms, and the site is easy to navigate.

United Ostomy Association

http://www.uoa.org

The United Ostomy Association (UOA) is a volunteer-based organization. It is dedicated to providing education, information, and support for individuals with an intestinal or urinary diversion. UOA is a member of the National Health Council, the National Digestive Diseases Information Clearinghouse, and the National Colorectal Cancer Roundtable, and is a charter member of the International Ostomy Association.

The site's intended audience is individuals with an ostomy or continent diversion. The UOA is in the process of forming a new support group specifically for people between the ages of 20 and 40. Information is current and accurate.

The site gives descriptions of ostomy procedures and different types of appliances. All major manufacturers are covered. Information is also given on local chapters and support groups for individuals and parents, insurance coverage selection, suppliers, and other ostomy sites, including links to the International Ostomy Association and the World Ostomy Resource.

The information covers many aspects, concerns, and questions a new ostomate may have. It provides an immense amount of information on different types of surgeries, appliances, and support groups.

The site is easy to use and graphically appealing.

Part IV

Negotiating the Health Care System

_____ Chapter 37

Long-Term Care Services

Ethel L. Mitty, PhD, RN

_____

This chapter is a good place to start for information on virtually all aspects of the long-term care (LTC) continuum and issues of interest to the older adult. The Web sites have been in existence long enough to have benefited from user feedback; all of them are easy to use and have an extensive system of linkages. Even for those who do not feel completely proficient in computer skills, professional and layperson, it is unlikely that information and access needs will be unmet. The sites were selected for their broad range of appeal and utility. Professionals from diverse disciplines (health care, law, social services), older adults, family members, surrogate decision makers, and guardians will find useful information in these sites, if only as a starting-off point. Among the sites, areas covered include housing and residential care options; home modification; elder abuse and fraud; retirement planning and LTC insurance; health facts and topics in clinical care; policy updates; end-of-life planning and care (hospice, palliative care); bereavement counseling; ombudsman services; domains of LTC (e.g., nursing homes, subacute care, assisted living); Medicare, Medicaid, and other government programs, including community-based services; general consumer information; and caregiver resources. Among all the sites, only one presents a portion of its information in Spanish; however, there are some links to other Web sites in other languages.

American Association for Retired Persons

http://www.aarp.org

The Web site of the American Association for Retired Persons (AARP) is updated frequently and primarily targeted to the well older adult. A lifestyle advocacy as well as a political action association, its Web site topics include AARP member services and discounts, research and reference sources, and information on computers, health and wellness, legislation, leisure and travel, money management, work options, and volunteer experiences. Overall, the content of the site is designed to encourage, inform, advise, and warn the older consumer about opportunities, resources, and hazards. For example, recent articles on the site addressed learning how to fix a hard drive after a computer crashes and warnings about the seductiveness of e-commerce to manage finances and investments. Access is also provided to *Modern Maturity,* the AARP magazine; many articles and features are made available on the site.

A feature on end-of-life resources and the search for a good death addressed the need for advance planning about treatment preferences and encouraged browsers to watch a PBS program on death and dying in America. The page provided linkages to related indexes on health and wellness, life transitions, Internet resources related to aging, and AARP grief and loss resources. These included a segment on reactions and commonly asked questions about coping with grief and loss, resources for professionals, a survivor's "guide" that addressed insurance, estate taxes, and housing, grief in the workplace, and the AARP Grief and Loss Programs. The Web site has a legal services network that provides information about the difference between a will and a living trust, suggests how to manage funeral expenses and arrangements, and offers AARP members a free 30-minute consultation with an attorney in the person's community (who meets AARP standards). The "Health and Wellness" and "Life Transitions" pages have extensive links to resources for caregivers. Although some of the services are available only to AARP members, the site is a good place to start for well elderly who are feeling somewhat overwhelmed by living alone in the face of potentially daunting health, emotional, and financial issues. Health professionals should become familiar with what this site has to offer because it has practical and thoughtful information for the older and not necessarily retired adult.

American Association of Homes and Services for the Aging

http://www.aahsa.org

This is the site of the American Association of Homes and Services for the Aging (AAHSA), the national association of nonprofit nursing homes, continuing care retirement communities (CCRC), assisted living residences, senior housing, and community service organizations for the elderly. Although the site is targeted to long-term care professionals and providers, it has an extensive and valuable repository of consumer information that is easily accessible for the older browser. The "Consumer Tips" pages, all of which can be downloaded, include "Choosing an Assisted Living Facility," "Finding the Right Nursing Home," "Home and Community-based Services," "Federally Funded Senior Housing," and "Selecting a CCRC." The site also provides a directory of accredited CCRCs, accreditation by virtue of the facility having met AAHSA standards. The Center for Medicare Education, a resource for public agencies and private organizations that provide consumer education about Medicare and Medicaid health plan options, could be of interest and value to beneficiaries who want to know more about their health care coverage options.

The fact that this Web site is directed toward health care professionals should not deter nurses from suggesting access to those clients who can effectively use the information to guide their quests and choices. Despite the fact that the site does not show a specific link to consumer information, the opening page of the site lists consumer information resources, as described above. The site also offers Web site links, but the information provided by this access is more efficiently accessed through the "Elderweb" and "Elderpage" sites (see separate entries). The "Research and Reference Link," a compendium of research papers produced by the association, would be least helpful to the average browser.

American Health Care Association

http://www.ahca.org

The American Health Care Association (AHCA) site primarily represents for-profit providers of long-term care services. The "Consumer Information" page, immediately accessible from a list of topics, is engaging and easy to peruse. After a brief description of AHCA's mission, information is given on nursing homes and subacute care, assisted living, and intermediate care facilities. Additional topics include a "consumer's guide" to nursing homes and assisted living, a family guide to making the transition to institutional care; myths and realities about nursing homes, LTC insurance, and Alzheimer's disease and related dementias. In addition, the reader can access Medline, get information about Medicare and managed care, and learn more about volunteering in the community.

The "Research and Data" information services can be helpful for the consumer who wants to know more about the impact of public policy on long-term care services. AHCA produces the annual *Facts and Trends Sourcebook* on nursing facilities, assisted living facilities, and subacute care that describes user characteristics, the services available, and utilization facts.

Assisted Living Federation of America

http://www.alfa.org

National Center for Assisted Living

http://www.ncal.org

These sites represent assisted living facilities' national organizations: the Assisted Living Federation of America (ALFA) and the National Center for Assisted Living (NCAL), an affiliate of the American Health Care Association (see separate entry). ALFA membership also includes continuing care retirement communities, independent living and other types of housing, and services for the elderly. Both sites describe assisted living, provide some facts about occupancy and services, and instruct the reader on how to get a list of residences. Each site has educational materials for the older person who is considering various housing options. ALFA-produced consumer education videos about the decision-making process of moving into an assisted living facility can be purchased through the online bookstore. Two documents on the ALFA site can be extremely useful: (1) the "Consumer Information Statement," which can help a prospective resident and family compare facilities, and (2) the "Model Admissions Agreement," which clearly specifies what a facility should include in an admission contract, such as what the facility will and will not provide, all costs, and discharge criteria.

The "Consumer Information" page of the NCAL site is an unfussy list of topics, each of which is thoroughly presented, accurate, and timely. The browser can go to a comprehensive description of assisted living, a guide to selecting an assisted living or residential care facility (i.e., services to look for), a by-state facility locator, and a 13-page article on long-term care insurance that is well written and very informative.

Sections of the article address if, when, and how much insurance to buy, services covered and not covered, complaints, cancellation, and a glossary of health insurance coverage terms.

Elderpage: Information for Older Persons and Families

http://www.aoa.dhhs.gov/elderpage.html

The federal government's Administration on Aging (AOA) "Elderpage" Web site, designed for health care professionals, older adults, and family members, gives links to virtually every aspect of aging, from housing options and mental health services to retirement planning and long-term care insurance. This is a user-friendly site, with current and accurate information about policy, regulations, and resources. The site provides information on the Aging Network and state and area agencies on aging and the LTC Ombudsman Program. Among the best features, and there are many good resources on this site, are the "Fact Sheets on Aging," the National Institute on Aging "Age Pages" (two- to four-page booklets mostly on health topics), and the "Eldercare Locator," a link to local support services and agencies throughout the United States, classified by region and type of service. A toll-free number is provided. The "Eldercare Locator" provides information about respite, finding help to remain independent, meals, transportation, housing options, home repair, legal service, and so on.

Several very informative health maintenance booklets that can be downloaded include "Talking With Your Doctor: A Guide for Older People", "Memory Exercises," and "My Medicines," a brochure from the Food and Drug Administration on using medications wisely. Links are available for housing concerns, such as home modification and repair, assisted living, shared housing, and government-assisted housing. Other links give information on elder abuse, fraud, women's health, Medicare, Alzheimer's disease, veterans' benefits, disaster recovery, unpaid family leave to take an elderly relative to a physician's appointment, legal rights and assistance, Social Security benefits, LTC insurance, electronic tax submission, and volunteer opportunities. One of the links is to AccessAmerica for Seniors (*www.seniors.gov*); the first page is "newsy" and updated every 2 or 3 days. From this page, one can get information about Medicare, choosing a nursing home, retirement planning and tax assistance, education and training, and travel and leisure. Unfortunately, as with most e-site publications, the material is available only in English. The information and linkage directions are easy to read and follow. As with virtually all sites that provide information on request, there is a statement about confidentiality.

Elderweb

http://www.elderweb.com

One of the oldest elder care sources on the Internet, "Elderweb" has fewer links than the AOA "Elderpage" (see separate entry), but is as comprehensive, current, and accurate. It supplies health care, financial, medical, policy, and research information to health care professionals, elders, and family members. The site is published by Karen Stevenson Brown, CPA, and is easy to use. The homepage lists the week's "Headlines" such as Medicare prescription drug coverage and finding reclaimed property and unclaimed assets, and "Coming Events," such as the Global Conference on Aging and the National Association of Professional Geriatric Care Managers Annual Conference, all of which can be opened for additional information.

Easy-to-access links go to sites on "Finance and Law," "Living Arrangements," "Associations and Agencies" (by region and topic or service provided), the "Eldercare Locator," and "Elderweb." The "Body and Soul" link offers information on elderly persons' physical needs, as well as the mental, social, and spiritual needs of the elderly and their caregivers. Users can select from a glossary of health and medical terms and common geriatric syndromes, including falls and incontinence. The incontinence page, for example, reports recent findings on incontinence and falls and provides links to articles, associations, and advice from physicians, nurses, and physical therapists. "Associations and Agencies" includes topics such as death and funerals, hospice care, vision and hearing, wellness, and nutrition. The information and link directions are easy to read and follow, especially because the print size can be increased to make reading easier.

Family Caregiver Alliance

http://www.caregiver.org

National Alliance for Caregiving

http://www.caregiving.org

National Family Caregivers Association

http://www.nfcacares.org

These Web sites are community-based nonprofit organizations that address the needs and interests of family members and friends providing long-term care at home. Each site offers low-key physical and mental health advice, encourages self-care and self-advocacy, and provides information on a range of long-term caregiving issues. The language and writing styles on the sites are undemanding.

The Family Caregiver Alliance (FCA) is the lead agency in California's system of Caregiver Resource Centers. To access information on caregiver services, users must first go to the *caregiver.org* "Resource Center" page. Once there, users can choose from topics of care, including behavior management strategies, community care options, conservatorship, advance directives, finding an attorney, hiring in-home help, and planning for incapacity. The site also provides links to other sources, such as the "Work/Eldercare" site.

The National Alliance for Caregiving (NAC) homepage (*www.caregiving.org*) is easier to peruse than the *caregiver.org* homepage and clearly lists the advice and resources provided. Users can go immediately to the "Caregiving Tips" page, which, while giving the reader a pep talk, also gives some advice for realistic goal setting and healthy assertiveness to demand correct and adequate information from health care professionals. Pages include summaries of reports and new products, a "Family Care Resource Connection," study and survey abstracts, a description of grassroots efforts to foster local caregiver support groups, and a "CareWizard" section.

The National Family Caregivers Association (NFCA) homepage (*www.nfcacares.org*) is a no-frills description of what the NFCA is and does. Among the three organizations, the NFCA speaks directly to the right of a caregiver to a reasonable quality of life achieved, in part, by taking charge of his or her own life. However, the site is cumbersome because some of the helpful information is considered a "service" and other material is listed under "Caregiver Tips." Failure to note where information is located could mean wasting time finding it again. The site is clearly dedicated to caregivers' well-being, from thrice-yearly upbeat messages to members to an intelligent list of suggestions on improving doctor/caregiver communications. The NFCA offers a bereavement kit available from the Web site. Links to aging-related resources are probably easier accessed via other sites.

Last Acts: A National Coalition to Improve Care and Caring at the End of Life

http://www.lastacts.org

The Last Acts homepage is easily negotiated. It begins with a very brief description of the Last Acts program and immediately offers users an array of information and resources, all of which are easily accessible. Reference to this site should be preceded by at least a modicum of understanding that the goal of Last Acts is to help individuals and organizations pursue better ways to care for the dying; the organization wholeheartedly supports palliative care as a holistic and humanistic way to provide the best quality of life until the end of life. The site provides cutting-edge information and expertise on a broad range of topics. Last Acts is a membership organization, with former First Lady Rosalynn Carter its honorary chair.

The late summer 2000 homepage included access to information on a hospice teen volunteer program, a book shop, an article from *Modern Maturity* (see American Association for Retired Persons entry) on end-of-life care, findings from a study about adolescents and loss, and an interactive questionnaire on views on end-of-life issues. In addition, an extensive resource directory listed national and state organizations and agencies concerned with chronic progressive disease, pain, hospice care, and dying, suggested further readings, and gave Internet resources. "Information for Families," accessed via the "Electronic Newsletter" page, defines and clarifies what palliative care is (i.e., it recognizes the spiritual needs of patient and family), directs the reader to the resource list, suggests questions a progressively ill person should ask his or her family, physician, and clergy, and talks about choices. A link to "Other Resources" guides selection by type of resource (i.e., hard copy, electronic, or audiovisual) and topic, such as adult day care, bereavement, finances, managed care, legal issues, and volunteering. Unfortunately, the Spanish-language version of "Precepts for Palliative Care" is not available on the site.

National Citizen's Coalition for Nursing Home Reform

http://www.nccnhr.org

The goal of the National Citizen's Coalition for Nursing Home Reform (NCCNHR) is to define, achieve, and maintain quality of care for people with long-term care needs in nursing homes and assisted living and board-and-care facilities. The NCCNHR is a high-profile consumer advocacy group active in public policy debate and resident rights and protection. The site is recommended for residents, family members, and others who want to be active participants in the discussion of critical issues of long-term care. The coalition has taken a position on minimum staffing standards in nursing homes and, through its publications, addressed how to get good care in a nursing home, the use of physical restraints, and guidelines to obtain legal advice. Links to the "Family Involvement" and "Citizen Groups" arms of the NCCNHR open the door to local action, such as "advocacy tips" and suggestions on how to change the culture of a nursing home.

Ombudspersons, key members of the NCCNHR, provide information on how to find a facility and educate residents and families about resident rights, quality of care surveys, and federal and state nursing home regulations. The site provides direct links to ombudsman offices in every state. The Ombudsman Resource Center is funded by the Administration on Aging (see separate entry) and managed by the NCCNHR to provide support, technical assistance, and training to ombudspersons. The homepage is straightforward; the links are easily accessed.

—————————————————— Chapter 38

Home Care Services

Georgia L. Narsavage, PhD, RN, CS

H ome care services increasingly have replaced hospital services for many patients. As the population in the United States has aged, millions of older adults now live with chronic illness, preferring to stay in their home setting as long as possible. Most problems may be managed in the home environment with appropriate support. Home care providers can help patients and their caregivers safely use equipment and related procedures, manage day-to-day living with disease and disability, and identify and respond to complications. The role of nurses and other professionals delivering care within the home setting includes components of assessment, direct care provision, and patient/family education.

Therapies such as nutrition and intravenous medications have become quite common in the home care setting. New equipment and procedures can be overwhelming for patients, particularly when the ability to learn is compromised by anxiety, depression, language barriers, low literacy, or sensory deficits. Problems arise when hospital discharge teaching does not transfer to the home environment, distractions are present, and no professional is readily available to help with problem-solving or to provide assurance that things are "going right." Patient coping and the availability of competent support from family members and friends influence the requirements for professional or custodial assistance at home.

Home care services can prevent unnecessary hospital admissions or emergency room visits and may help patients and caregivers to recognize complications before a crisis occurs. Such services may be needed to help with newly prescribed equipment or procedures; and difficulty with activities of daily living (ADLs) such as bathing or instrumental activities of daily living (IADLs) such as cooking. Disruptive family dynamics, alcohol or drug abuse, dementia, mental illness, and severe anxiety or depression can seriously affect the ability of patients and families to manage at home. An understanding of what websites can offer should help guide families toward sources of information and available contacts.

Patients receiving intermittent home care services usually are over age 65 and are primarily reimbursed by the Medicare program, which was designed to cover acute episodes of illness, not chronic or maintenance care. Medicare regulations are highly specific and reimburse only care that is skilled or delivered by a skilled professional, is intermittent, is covered by a physician's order, and is delivered to patients who remain homebound. Agencies certified by Medicare to provide home care may be for-profit or nonprofit in nature and may be hospital-based or freestanding. Home medical equipment and home pharmacy companies deliver, maintain, and instruct in the use of medically necessary equipment, such as oxygen, nebulizers, and ventilators, and pharmaceuticals such as inhaled and intravenous solutions. Although the major focus of these companies is on products and equipment, teaching safe use is an essential component. Caregivers need information on the selection of home care services, finances, provisions for emergencies, family support services, counseling, help in managing the stress and emotional demands of caregiving, and means to provide continuity after formal home care services have ended.

There are four national home health associations that can be accessed to assist consumers in obtaining up-to-date answers to their questions. One of these, the American Home Care Association, was formed in December 2000 when the Home Care Association of America merged with the American Federation of Home Care Providers, a trade association. Additionally the website for the American Association of Retired Persons (AARP) is an excellent source for updated home care services information on its documents section titled "AARP Research: Health and Long-Term Care." The links from these websites are extensive, including national government and state agencies, but one should note that there might be bias in sites that present commercial products and services.

American Association for Home Care

http://www.aahomecare.org

A merger of home care providers supports this association website for consumers of home care services. It represents over 1,000 home care provider members who offer home care services, medical equipment and supplies, and variety of therapy/rehabilitation services.

This site states that its mission is to promote consumer access to home health care, with links to its partner: The Caregivers Advisory Panel (TCAP), a national panel of family caregiver market research volunteers. Sections include the Resource Directory, Government Relations, Meetings & Education, Products & Services, and Press Releases. The intended audience is AAHC members and consumer caregivers. Information is accurate and timeliness is indicated by the weekly update on the press releases available to consumers. Phone and e-mail contact information is provided.

Some of the site's best features are that it communicates home care legislation and provides a regulatory advocacy network, along with educational program information and Medicare reimbursement assistance for AAHC members. The AAHomecare Online Resource Directory is easily searched by keyword or category. Links to caregiver support sites with the Caregivers Advisory Panel is an opportunity for consumers to provide feedback to provider organizations through the Caregivers homepage link *http://www.caregiversadvisorypanel.com* or via toll-free telephone (877)595-6227.

The site itself is a link to useful caregiver sites, but the funding sources are not explicit. It was formed by a merger of commercial agencies: the Health Industry Distributors Association's Home Care Division (HIDA Home Care), Home Health Services & Staffing Association (HHSSA), and the National Association for Medical Equipment Services (NAMES). The website for AAHC is primarily organized for its member agencies, so there are frequent limitations to Members Only on the site. Consumers may not see the informative nature of the caregiver information and benefit of providing opinions that can affect policy decisions. Information is in English only. Although it is not a sophisticated website, the legislative focus serves a useful purpose. Navigation is not difficult.

American Association of Retired Persons (AARP): Research on Health & Long-Term Care

http://research.aarp.org/health/list.html

The American Association of Retired Persons (AARP) is a national nonprofit organization designed to improve the lives of older Americans. It has 30 million members. This site provides information on issues of interest to individuals over age 50, with online access to the journal, other publications and activities of AARP. AARP section links include Health & Long-Term Care, Economic Security & Work, Independent Living, Consumer Issues, Demographics & References, Research Digest, Ageline Database, and Public Policy Institute. The site is frequently updated.

Important features are the extensive list of documents of interest to consumers, including state profiles and resources and in-depth reports such as "Assuring the Quality of Home Care: The Challenge of Involving the Consumer."

Examining the extensive information offered may be frustrating as consumers attempt to find the most important documents. Information is in English only. This is a sophisticated website that is frequently updated. Consumers should have no difficulty navigating the site.

American Home Care Association, Inc.

http://www.americanhca.com

This association website was developed following the merger of the Home Care Association of America with the American Federation of Home Care Providers, Inc. trade association to provide education, assistance to home care agencies, and national representation for home health care services. AHCA states that its purpose is to provide assistance to home care providers and organizations that serve home care providers. The intended audience is home care agencies and their patients, as well as organizations providing services to home care agencies.

The web page did not include the date of the last update. Timeliness of reports was not clear but Web site update followed the association merger date of December 2000. Accuracy is enhanced in the provider list of home care agencies via a feedback link, so that inaccuracies and updated agency information can be reported directly to AHCA.

The site provides easily understood news releases on home health, presenting issues of interest to consumers attempting to understand legislation and policies affecting home care service. One useful aspect of this website is external links that enable an easy search of "Thomas" for contacting the U.S. congressional representatives and for information on the U.S. Department of Health and Human Services *http:// www.hhs.gov/agencies*, as well as internal links to State Associations for Home Care. The "Locate a Health Care Provider" link on the home page of AHCA is a comprehensive and easy-to-search list of agencies by geography.

Some features such as "NewsServe" are usually limited to members and not available to consumers. The uninitiated may not be able to differentiate the information available to all viewers from member service information. This may be a result of the need to continue the trade association information along with consumer information. Information is in English only. The site has a relatively simple appearance making news updates easy to read. Links require several steps until the consumer information is presented.

Home Care Association of America (HCAA)

http://www.hcaa-homecare.com

This is an association website representing freestanding home health care services as small-business agencies and home-bound patients/ families. HCAA states that its purpose is to provide a forum for freestanding home care service agencies to understand current policy issues and to advocate for home care consumers. The web page includes the date of the last update. Accuracy of reports was not clear as the website update was greater than 3 months at the time of review.

The site provides easily understood news releases on legislation and policies affecting home care service. One useful aspect of this website is the easily searched "Contact your Rep" for contacting congressional representatives. PPS Clinical Pathways provides a useful link to layman's explanations of clinical specialty areas in home care to assist consumers in understanding what services could be provided in a home setting (*http://www.clinicalpathways.homepage.com/ SpecialtyPathways.htm*).

The editorial pages include exclamatory remarks that must be examined carefully for bias. Information is in English only.This site has a relatively simple appearance that is easy to use.

Home Care in Cyberspace

http://www.ptct.com/cyber_industry.html

These sites are lists of links to web sites of individual home care agencies and home health care organizations. They highlight agencies and organizations who have supported the sponsors. The sites are designed to be identified by major search engines when consumers are looking for information on home care services. Michelle Scott Hamilton is the founder and president of USA Homecare. Patient Care Technologies manages the Home Care in Cyberspace site. It is a private company that provides information services and administrative support for agencies, including homecare services. Accuracy may be influenced by the profit-seeking motivation but the information is updated frequently and appears timely.

The breadth and depth of information on the sites are useful, as long as potential bias is considered. Links to updated Medline reviews of home care information provides access to accurate professional healthcare information. Keep in mind that the for-profit sponsorship means the authors are attempting to sell their product. Information is in English only. The site provides easy-to-use links to multiple websites, but the variety of information may be overwhelming to the consumer.

Home Care Online

http://www.nahc.org

This website represents the interests of home care services and hospices, including corporations, state home care associations, medical equipment suppliers, and educational institutions. It is sponsored by the National Association for Home Care (NAHC).

The NAHC website has a threefold purpose: 1) to provide members with professional advice and assistance on administrative and legal issues; 2) to distribute information to consumers and the media that increases knowledge and acceptance of home care and hospice services; and 3) to provide support for families and other caregivers. The intended audience is consumers and association home care member agencies.

This is a good starting-point for consumers because it provides a broad-based source of information on home care services. It is worthwhile to refer consumers to this site because the information is accurate, timely, and frequently updated. The NAHC provides a comprehensive source of consumer information, which is accessed by a "consumer" button on the homepage. The Consumer Information section of this website provides online links to general topics and information on patient's rights and payment practices. (Access directly with *http:// www.nahc.org/Consumer/coninfo.html*). The best feature is a consumer guide on "How to Choose a Home Care Provider." It can be purchased in hard copy and is also available as full text online. Other useful information is a home care and hospice agency locator and an easily searchable list of State Resources, with contact phone numbers.

As a trade association keep in mind that information could be biased. Providing information in other languages such as Spanish would have been valuable. State resources do not include links to websites. This is an appealing website, well-organized and easily understood.

USA Homecare.com

Http://www.usahomecare.com/hotlist.htm

Visiting Nurse Associations of America (VNAA)

http://www.vnaa.org

The VNAA links over 200 not-for-profit home health care agencies in 40 states to provide a strong network for growth and development. The site is designed to be accessed easily by both agency members and consumers. Its purpose is to support delivery of home care services by enhancing communication between and among agencies and consumers in order to fulfill the VNAA mission as an essential health care service in the community. The high standards of the VNAA result in an informative, accurate, and current source of information for the consumer.

Best features include both Home Care Resources and Caregiver Information sections. The Caregiver's Handbook is available online or can be ordered in hard copy.

No critical weaknesses were noted although more information in other languages would be valuable. The site is easily read and navigated by even novice internet users. Frequent requests for donations on multiple pages can be viewed negatively by those interested in obtaining information quickly. Information is in English only.

Chapter 39

Understanding Medical Jargon

Sarah P. Farrell, PhD, RN, CS

O ne of the biggest obstacles to patient empowerment may have to do with language. What is the nurse or doctor talking about? This chapter represents an effort to provide the consumer with the tools to understand the very basic terminology used by health care professionals.

European Commission Glossary

http://allserv.rug.ac.be/~rvdstich/eugloss/welcome.html

This is a multilingual glossary of technical and popular medical terms in nine European languages (Dutch, French, German, English, Spanish, Italian, Portuguese, Greek, and Danish). The project is the result of a European Commission directive to develop and standardize full-information patient package inserts, written in lay language, for some 6,000 medicinal preparations. The project began in 1988 and was completed in 1991. It was executed by the Heymans Institute of Pharmacology and the Mercator School, Department of Applied Linguistics, in Belgium.

The site was last updated several months prior to our review. The final basic English list consists of 1,830 terms. Translators were given a fair amount of freedom in proposing the deletion of terms for which popular equivalents are redundant, the scientific term having become perfectly intelligible to the average lay reader. The site is straightforward and easy to use. The reading level is average to above average.

The design of the site is practical and professional. Users choose a particular language, then scan an alphabetical list to find the definition of a term. A technical and a popular medical equivalent are provided for each term.

The Merck Manual—Home Edition

http://www.merckhomeedition.com

According to Copernic 2000, a meta-search engine, "We've praised the online Merck manuals in the past. The latest one, the Merck Manual of Medical Information—Home Edition, is even better because it translates the jargon from the professional edition into language the rest of us can understand."

The site is a free online version of *The Merck Manual*, the textbook of medicine most widely used by health care professionals in the United States. The *Home Edition* transforms the language of the professional version into commonly used English while retaining vital information on diseases, diagnoses, and prevention and treatment options. The sponsor is Merck Co., a manufacturer of pharmaceuticals and other health care products. Consumers are the target audience, but this is also a nice resource for students and practitioners from different disciplines. Users can search through the site's table of contents to find information on diseases, drugs, and medical tests.

The information is not watered down, so the reading level would be considered above average. However, from a consumer's perspective, the complex material is made comprehensible. The site loads quickly, is easy to navigate, and is graphically appealing. Buttons and icons are easy to use.

Chapter 40

Medical Devices

Sarah P. Farrell, Phd, RN, CS

Τhis chapter covers U.S. and international Web sites related to medical devices. Because of the nature of the topic, the sites are technical and may be difficult and inappropriate for the average consumer. Included are the homepages of government agencies, starting with the U.S. Food and Drug Administration and extending to the top sites for government agencies in Australia and the United Kingdom. The sites were selected for their accuracy, completeness, and professionalism. They feature easy search-and-find functions. Medical devices can be anything from thermometers to artificial hearts to at-home pregnancy test kits (Federal Food, Drug and Cosmetic Act, Section 201).

Food and Drug Administration, United States

http://www.fda.gov

This is the main site for the U.S. Food and Drug Administration (FDA). The FDA is one of the nation's oldest and most respected consumer protection agencies. Its mission is to promote and protect the public health by helping safe and effective products reach the market in a timely way and by monitoring products for continued safety after they are in use. The site is sponsored by the FDA's Office of Public Affairs, U.S. Department of Health and Human Services. The page is updated at least weekly.

This comprehensive site is useful to consumers who are interested in finding out the status of a specific medical device. It gives volumes of technical information, including regulations and manufacturers' specifications. This is one of the most current and accurate sites on this topic.

The site is easy to navigate and graphically appealing. The special "Kids" link includes the "Parents' Corner," "Teen Scene," Yorick, the bionic skeleton, and a delightful medical device learning tool.

Food and Drug Administration (U.S.): Center for Devices and Radiological Health

http://www.fda.gov/cdrh/index.html

The Center for Devices and Radiological Health (CDRH) site is a subsite of the FDA homepage (see separate entry). Their mission is protecting the public health by providing reasonable assurance of the safety and effectiveness of medical devices and by eliminating unnecessary human exposure to radiation emitted from electronic products. The CDRH is responsible for regulating medical devices and radiation-emitting products.

For consumers, there are easy links to the following categories: "Popular Items," "Interacting with CDRH," "Special Interest," "Pre-market," "Post-market," "Radiation Health," "Topic Index," and the FDA homepage.

Medical Devices Agency, United Kingdom

http://www.medical-devices.gov.uk

This site is sponsored by the Medical Devices Agency, an arm of the British government charged with safeguarding public health by working with users, manufacturers, and legislators to ensure that medical devices meet appropriate standards of safety, quality, and performance and that they comply with relevant directives of the European Union. The purpose of this site is to provide the standards online. The text language is technical and may be difficult for the average consumer.

Therapeutic Goods Administration, Australia

http://www.health.gov.au/tga/devices/devices.htm.

This is another international site, sponsored by an agency of the Australian government. Information is technical and may be difficult for the average consumer.

Chapter 41

Health Insurance

Ruth Chasek

Obtaining and financing health insurance can be a major health problem that most health care professionals aren't prepared to address. It also requires some knowledge of the health system. What is an HMO? What is a PPO? How do I know which plan lets me choose my own physician? Working families may be presented with a bewildering menu of health insurance choices at work. Unemployed, low income, or self-employed individuals and families may have no health insurance or inadequate insurance. The sites listed below offer a basic primer on the health insurance system, and ways to choose the best option for your needs.

Check Up on Health Insurance Choices

and

Choosing and Using a Health Plan

http://www.ahrq.gov/consumer
(look under "Health Plans")

These two online brochures are part of the consumer section of the U.S. Agency for Health Research and Quality Web site. Both brochures provide a clear and understandable description of health insurance options for consumers. They describe traditional fee-for-service plans, HMOs, Medicare, Medicaid, disability insurance, and long term care insurance. Lists of questions to ask of various types of health plans are included, as well as a glossary of insurance terms ("Understanding Health Insurance Terms"). There are also a checklist of important features in a health plan and a worksheet for determining the best buy. The Agency for Health Research and Quality (AHRQ) is part of the United States Government. Its mission is to develop research-based information on health care outcomes, quality, cost, use, and access. Its consumer health section is an excellent source of health information. It is not comprehensive, but includes consumer versions of AHRQ clinical practice guidelines on a wide range of diseases and conditions, which were developed by panels of health care experts. Much of the information is available in Spanish and English. Unfortunately, the health insurance information is not available in Spanish, but perhaps it will be in the future. Information is presented on a simple-to-understand level and is easy to find.

Insure Kids Now: Linking the Nation's Children to Health Insurance

http://www.insurekidsnow.gov

Insure Kids Now is a national campaign to link the approximately 10 million uninsured children in the United States to free or low cost health insurance. It is sponsored by the Health Resources and Services Agency of the U.S. Department of Health and Human Services. Most states have programs to provide free or low cost health insurance to children and teens 18 years old or younger whose families earn up to $34,100 annually (for a family of four). A visitor to the site can click on his or her state, which will provide a link to that state's child health insurance program. Eligibility and contact information is included. This site is attractive, colorful, and easy to use. The language is simple and direct, and appropriate for consumers of any educational background. Calling the toll-free number 1-877-KIDS NOW is another way to access this information. This Web site is completely bilingual in Spanish and English.

Appendix

ALPHABETICAL INDEX OF WEB SITES

Web Site	Language other than English	Page number
Alcoholics Anonymous *http://alcoholics-anonymous.org*	Spanish and French	63
American Academy of Allergy, Asthma, and Immunology *http://www.aaai.org*		26
American Academy of Pain Management *http://www.aapainmanage.org*		128
American Academy of Sleep Medicine *http://www.aasmnet.org*		144
American Association for Home Care *http://www.aahomecare.org*		188
American Association for Retired Persons *http://www.aarp.org*		177
Health and Long-Term Care *http://research.aarp.org/health/list.html*		189
American Association of Homes and Services for the Aging *http://www.aahsa.org*		178
American Bar Association Against Domestic Violence *http://www.abanet.org/domviol/home.html*		57
American Botanical Council *http://www.herbalgram.org*		45
American Cancer Society *http://www.cancer.org*	some Spanish	33
Prostate Cancer Resource Center *http://www3.cancer.org/cancerinfo* (select "Prostate Cancer")		138
American Council on Exercise *http://www.acefitness.org*		82
American Diabetes Association *http://www.diabetes.org*	Spanish	49
American Dietetic Association *http://www.eatright.org*		54

Web Site	Language other than English	Page number
American Foundation for Urologic Disease *http://www.afud.org*		113
American Health Care Association *http://www.ahca.org*		179
American Heart Association *http://www.americanheart.org*		91
American Heart Association: Take Wellness to Heart Campaign *http://www.women.americanheart.org*		93
American Home Care Association *http://www.americanhca.org*		189
American Medical Association *www.ama-assn.org*		7
American Society of Clinical Oncology *http://www.asco.org*		34
American Stroke Association *http://www.strokeassociation.org*		155
Assisted Living Federation of America *http://www.alfa.org*		180
Association of Occupational and Environmental Clinics *http://www.aoec.org*		76
Babycenter—Immunizations: What You Need to Know About Them *http://www.babycenter.com/refcap/95.html*		110
BirthPlan.com *http://www.birthplan.com*	Spanish	133
Bladder Control for Women *http://www.niddk.nih.gov/health/urolog/* *uibcw/index.htm*	Spanish	114
The Body: An AIDS and HIV Information Resource *http://www.thebody.com*	Spanish	106
Cancer Care *http://www.cancercare.org*	Spanish	35

Web Site	Language other than English	Page number
Cancer Education *http://www.cancereducation.com*		36
Cancerfacts *http://www.cancerfacts.com*		36
Cancernet *http://www.cancernet.nci.nih.gov*		37
Cancer-Prostate.com *http://www.cancer-prostate.com*		140
Caregivers.com *http://www.caregivers.com*		68
Caring for Someone with AIDS at Home *http://www.hivatis.org/caring*		107
CBS Healthwatch by Medscape *http://www.healthwatch.medscape.com*		163
CDC Guide to Caring for Someone with AIDS at Home *http://www.hivatis.org/caring*		107
Center for Devices and Radiological Health *http://www.fda.gov/cdrh/index.html*		196
Centers for Disease Control and Prevention *http://www.cdc.gov*	some Spanish	4
Check Up on Health Insurance Choices, and Choosing and Using a Health Plan *http://www.ahrq.gov/consumer* (look under Health Plans)		197
Childbirth.org *http://www.childbirth.org*		134
Children's Defense Fund *http://www.childrensdefense.org*		39
Children's Environmental Health Network *http://www.cehn.org*		77
Children's Health Information Network *http://www.tchin.org*		94
Children with Diabetes *http://www.childrenwithdiabetes.com*		50

Web Site	Language other than English	Page number
Choice in Dying *http://www.choices.org*		70
Cocaine Anonymous World Services Online *http://www.ca.org*	French	63
Complications in Spinal-Cord Injury *http://rehab.chungnam.ac.kr/english/ question/sci/2.html*		
Convatec Connection: Your Online Connection to Quality Information on Ostomy, Wound, and Skin Care *http://www.convatec.com*	German, French, Italian, and Spanish	173
Cure Paralysis Now *http://www.cureparalysis.org*		151
DadsWorld.com *http://www.dadsworld.com*		134
Death and Dying *http://death.net*	some Spanish	71
The Diabetes Mall *http://www.diabetesnet.com*		50
Disability-Specific Web Site *http://www.disserv.stu.umn.edu/disability*		125
Dr. Greene's Housecalls *http://www.drgreene.com/immunizations.asp*		111
Drug Addiction Rehabilitation Institute *http://www.innovativetreatment.org*		64
Eastern Paralyzed Veterans Association *http://www.epva.org*	Spanish	151
Elderpage: Information for Older Persons and Families *http://www.aoa.dhhs.gov/elderpage.html*		181
Elderweb *http://www.elderweb.com*		182
Empowering Caregivers *http://www.care-givers.com*		68

Web Site	Language other than English	Page number
Environmental Protection Agency: Concerned Citizens Resources *http://www.epa.gov/epapages/epahome/citizen.htm*		78
European Commission Glossary *http://allserv.rug.ac.be/~rvdstich/eugloss/welcome.html*	Dutch, French, German Spanish, Italian Portuguese, Greek, and Danish	193
Evergreen Health Care Family Maternity Center *http://www.evergreenhealthcare.org/maternity/questions.asp*		135
Exercise and Your Heart: A Guide to Physical Activity *http://www.nih.gov/health/exercise/index.htm*		83
Facts About Incontinence *http://www.nafc.org*		114
Family Caregiver Alliance *http://www.caregiver.org*		182
Family Peace Project: Medical College of Wisconsin *http://www.family.mcw.edu/familypeaceproject.htm*		58
Family Violence Prevention Fund *http://www.fvpf.org*		59
Farm-A-Syst Home-A-Syst: Help Yourself to a Healthy Home *http://www.uwex.edu/homeasyst*	some Spanish	79
Fatigue: How to Know When to See a Doctor *http://www.cnn.com/health/9909/21/lack.of.energy*		145
Fetal Alcohol Syndrome Assistance and Training *http://home.golden.net/~fasat*		64

Web Site	Language other than English	Page number
Fibromyalgia *http://www.nursece.com/onlinecourses/908.html*		145
Fitness Overview: Medem.com *http://www.medem.com* (click on "Medical Library," then "Fitness and Nutrition," then "Fitness Overview")		83
Food and Drug Administration *http://www.fda.gov*		195
FDA Consumer Drug Information Page *http://www.fda.gov/cder/consumerinfo*		15
FDA Information for Consumers *http://www.fda.gov/opacom/morecons.html*		15
Foodfit.com *http://www.foodfit.com*		55
Funeral.com *http://www.funeral.com*		71
Genetic Alliance *http://geneticalliance.org*	links to Spanish information	86
Genetics Education Center *http://www.kumc.edu/gec*		87
Global Neurologic Web sites *http://www.neuro.onnet.co.kr/links.html*	Korean	125
GriefNet *http://www.griefnet.org*		71
Health and Human Services Pages for Kids *http://www.hhs.gov/kids*	some Spanish	40
Health-Center.com Pharmacy *http://www1.health-center.com/pharmacy*		16
Healthfinder *http://www.healthfinder.gov*	some Spanish	5
HealthWeb *http://healthweb.org*		5
Heart Failure Online *http://www.heartfailure.org*	Spanish	95

Web Site	Language other than English	Page number
Heart Information Network *http://www.heartinfo.com*	some Spanish	96
HeartPoint *http://www.heartpoint.com*		97
The Hemlock Society *http://www.hemlock.org*		72
The Herpes Zone *http://www.herpeszone.com*		141
HIV InSite *http://www.hivinsite.ucsf.edu*		107
Hollister Inc. *http://www.hollister.com*	some Portuguese and Spanish	173
Home Care Association of America (HCAA) *http://www.hcaa-homecare.com*		190
Home Care in Cyberspace *http://www.ptct.com/cyber_industry.html*		191
Home Care Online *http://www.nahc.org*		192
Hospice Net: Death and Dying, Caregiving, and Grief *http://www.hospicenet.org*		73
Human Genome Project Information *http://www.ornl.gov/hgmis*		87
Immunizations: What You Need to Know *http://www.aap.org/family/vaccine.htm*		111
InfoMIN: Medical Information Network for Chronic Pain, CFS, FMS, and Other Medical Resources *http://www2.rpa.net/~lrandall/index.html*		129
Insulin Pumpers *http://www.insulin-pumpers.org*		51
Insure Kids Now: Linking the Nation's Children to Health Insurance *http://www.insurekidsnow.gov*	Spanish	198

Web Site	Language other than English	Page number
The Interactive Pregnancy Calendar *http://www.parentsplace.com/pregnancy/ calendar*		135
International Travel and Health: Vaccination Requirements and Health Advice (WHO) *http://www.who.int/ith*	French	158
International Travel Medicine Clinic *http://www.hsc.unt.edu/patientcare/itmc/ travel.htm*		159
Internet Mental Health *http://www.mentalhealth.com/p.html*	5 languages	120
Iwannaknow.org: Answers to Your Questions About Teen Sexual Health and STD Prevention *http://www.iwannaknow.org*		142
Johns Hopkins Heart Health: Patient Information *http://www.jhbmc.jhu.edu/cardiology/rehab/ patientinfo.html*		98
Joslin Diabetes Center *http://www.joslin.org*		52
Juvenile Diabetes Foundation International: The Diabetes Research Foundation *http://www.jdf.org*		52
La Leche League International *http://www.lalecheleague.org*	Spanish and Italian	30
Last Acts: A National Coalition to Improve Care and Caring at the End of Life *http://www.lastacts.org*		184
Links 2 Go: Death and Dying *http://www.links2go.com/topic/ Death_and_Dying*		73
Mayday Pain Project *http://www.painandhealth.org*		129
MayoClinic.com *http://www.mayoclinic.com*		6, 17

Web Site	Language other than English	Page number
MayoClinic.com: Heart and Blood Vessels Center *http://www.mayoclinic.com/home?id=3.1.9*		99
Medela *http://www.medela.com*		30
Medem *http://www.medem.com*		7
Medical Devices Agency, United Kingdom *http://www.medical-devices.gov.uk*		196
Medication Information Index *http://www.cheshire-med.com/services/ pharm/medindex.html*		17
MEDLINEplus *http://www.medlineplus.gov*	some Spanish	8, 17
MEDLINEplus: Exercise/Physical Fitness Section *http://www.nlm.nih.gov/medlineplus/ exercisephysicalfitness.html*		84
Mended Hearts Inc. *http://www.mendedhearts.org*		101
Mental Help Net *http://mentalhelp.net*		121
Mentalwellness.com: The Online Resource for Schizophrenia and Other Mental Health Information *http://www.mentalwellness.com*		122
The Merck Manual—Home Edition *http://www.merckhomeedition.com*		194
Minnesota Center Against Violence and Abuse *http://www.mincava.umn.edu*		59
Nanny's Place: Breastfeeding *http://www.moonlily.com/breastfeed*		31
Narconon—Reducing the Drug Problem *http://www.narconon.org*		65

Web Site	Language other than English	Page number
National Alliance for Caregiving *http://www.caregiving.org*		182
National Association on HIV Over Fifty *http://www.hivoverfifty.org*		69
National Center for Assisted Living *http://www.ncal.org*		180
National Center for Complementary and Alternative Medicine *http://www.nccam.nih.gov*	some Spanish	46
National Center for Education in Maternal and Child Health *www.ncemch.org*		41
National Citizen's Coalition for Nursing Home Reform *http://www.nccnhr.org*		184
National Coalition Against Domestic Violence *http://ncadv.org*		60
National Family Caregivers Association *http://www.nfcacares.org*		183
National Headache Foundation *http://www.headaches.org*		126
National Heart, Lung, and Blood Institute: Cardiovascular Information for Patients and the General Public *http://www.nhlbi.nih.gov/health/public/heart/index.htm*	some Spanish	102
National Human Genome Research Institute *http://www.nhgri.nih.gov*		88
National Institute of Child Health and Human Development *http://www.nichd.nih.gov*		42
National Institute of Drug Addiction: Principles of Drug Addiction Treatment *http://www.nida.nih.gov/PODAT/PODATindex.html*		65
National Institute of Mental Health *http://www.nimh.nih.gov*	some Spanish	123

Web Site	Language other than English	Page number
National Institute of Neurological Disorders and Stroke *http://www.ninds.nih.gov*		127, 156
National Institute on Aging Age Page, Medicines: Use Them Safely *http://www.aoa.dhhs.gov/aoa/pages/ agepages/medicine.html*		18
National Resource Center for Health and Safety in Child Care *http://nrc.uchsc.edu*		42
National Sleep Foundation *http://www.sleepfoundation.org*		146
National Spinal Cord Injury Association *http://www.spinalcord.org*		152
National Stroke Association *http://www.stroke.org*		156
National Women's Health Information Center *http://www.4women.org* or *http://www.4women.gov*	some Spanish	146, 164
National Women's Health Network *http://www.womenshealthnetwork.org*		165
National Women's Health Resource Center *http://www.healthywomen.org*		166
Neurogenic Bowel Management in Adults with Spinal Cord Injury *http://www.pva.org/pubsandproducts/ pvapubs/BowelProfessional.htm*		116
Neurogenic Bowel: What You Should Know *http://www.pva.org/sci/pubs/ consumerbowelmain.htm*		116
New York Online Access to Health *http://www.noah-health.org*	completely bilingual: English/ Spanish	10, 55

Web Site	Language other than English	Page number
NOAH (New York Online Access to Health) *http://www.noah-health.org*	completely bilingual: English/ Spanish	10, 55
Not-2-Late.Com: The Emergency Contraception Website *http://ec.princeton.edu*	Spanish, French	18
The Nursing Lounge *http://www.parentingweb.com/lounge/ lounge_index.htm*		31
Nutrition Navigator: A Rating Guide to Nutrition Web Sites *http://www.Navigator.tufts.edu*		55
Office of Rare Diseases, National Institutes of Health *http://rarediseases.info.nih.gov/ord/*		88
Oncolink *http://www.oncolink.com*		38
Online Mendelian Inheritance in Man: National Center for Biotechnology Information *http://www.ncbi.nlm.nih.gov/omim*		88
OSHA's Worker Page *http://www.osha.gov/as/opa/worker/ index.html*		80
Pain.com *http://www.pain.com*		130
Pain Medicine and Palliative Care *http://www.wehealny.org/services/pain/ index.html*		74
Partnership for Caring: America's Voices for the Dying *http://www.partnershipforcaring.org*		74
Pediatric Pain *http://is.dal.ca/%7Epedpain/pedpain.html*		131
Pets Are Loving Support *http://www.sonic.net/~pals*		108

Web Site	Language other than English	Page number
Planned Parenthood *http://www.plannedparenthood.org*	Spanish version of *Teenwire*	27
Precious Aromatherapy *http://www.aromatherapy.com*		47
Pregnancy and Exercise *http://lifematters.com/medicalinfo.html*		135
Pregnancy and HIV *http://www.hcfa.gov/hiv*		136
Pregnancy Bedrest *http://armstrong.son.wisc.edu/~son/bedrest*		136
ProMoM: Promotion of Mother's Milk Inc. *http://promom.org*		32
Quit4life *http://www.quit4life.com*	completely bilingual: English/ French	149
Quitnet *http://www.quitnet.org*		149
Resolve: The National Infertility Association *http://www.resolve.org*		118
Restless Legs Syndrome Foundation *http://www.rls.org*		147
Rick Mendosa's Diabetes Directory *http://www.mendosa.com/diabetes.htm*		53
Royal Adelaide Hospital Sexually Transmitted Disease Service *http://www.stdservices.on.net*		142
RxList *http://www.rxlist.com*		18
Senior Cyborgs *http://www.online96.com/seniors*		69
SkinWound.com *http://www.skinwound.com*		171

Web Site	Language other than English	Page number
Social Issues and Social Services: Death and Dying *http://www.mel.lib.mi.us/social/ SOC-death.html*		74
Society for Women's Health Research *http://www.womens-health.org*		168
Soyouwanna.com *http://soyouwanna.com/site/syws/quit/ quit.html*		150
Spinal Cord Injury—For Your Information *http://www.tbi-sci.org/scifyi*		153
Spinal Cord Injury Information Network *http://www.spinalcord.uab.edu*	Spanish	153
Spinal Cord Injury Ring *http://www.tbi-sci.org/sciring*		153
Stayhealthy.com *http://www.stayhealthy.com*		123
Taking Care of Your Bowels: The Basics *http://www.djepson.wiredup.com/ bowel1.html*		116
The Talarian Index *http://www.stat.washington.edu/TALARIA/ talaria0/TALARIA.html*		131
The Teen Pregnancy and Parenting Place *http://www.hometown.aol.com/mnn1121*		136
Teenshealth *http://www.teenshealth.org*		24
Therapeutic Goods Administration, Australia *http://www.health.gov.au/tga/devices/ devices.htm*		196
Thrive Online *http://thriveonline.oxygen.com*		143
Fitness Section *http://thriveonline.oxygen.com/fitness*		85
Travelers' Health (CDC) *http://www.cdc.gov/travel*	Spanish and Portuguese	160

Web Site	Language other than English	Page number
Travel Health Online *http://www.tripprep.com*		159
Travel Medicine Program, Health Canada *http://www.hc-sc.gc.ca/hpb/lcdc/osh/* *mp_e.html*	French	160
United Ostomy Association *http://www.uoa.org*		174
Urinary Incontinence: Embarrassing but Treatable *http://www.familydoctor.org/healthfacts/189/* *index.html*		115
USA Homecare.com *http://www.usahomecare.com/hotlist.htm*		192
U.S. Consumer Gateway: Health *http://www.consumer.gov/health.htm*	some other languages	11
U.S. Environmental Protection Agency Concerned Citizens Resources *http://www.epa.gov/epapages/epahome/* *citizen.htm*		78
U.S. Food and Drug Administration *http://www.fda.gov*		195
Center for Devices and Radiological Health *http://www.fda.gov/cdrh/index.html*		196
Visiting Nurse Associations of America *http://www.vnaa.org*		192
WebMD Health *http://mywebmd.com*		17
Weight-Control Information Network *http://www.niddk.nih.gov/health/nutrit/* *win.htm*		56
What Would Happen If We Stopped Vaccinations? *http://www.cdc.gov/nip/publications/fs/gen/* *WhatIfStop.htm*		112

Web Site	Language other than English	Page number
Women's Health Interactive *http://www.womens-health.com*	Some German in "Gynecological Health Center" section	169
Women's Health/Violence Against Women: Medem.com *http://www.medem.com* (click on "Medical Library," then "Women's Health," then "Violence Against Women")		61
World Health Organization *http://www.who.org*	Spanish and French	
Division of Child Health and Development *http://www.who.int/chd*		43
International Travel and Health *http://www.who.int/ith*		158
Wound Care Information Network *http://www.medicaledu.com/wndguide.htm*		172
The Yoga Group: Yoga for HIV/AIDS *http://www.yogagroup.org*		108
Youth Resource *http://www.youthresource.com*		109

Index

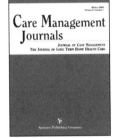

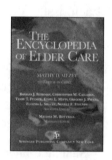

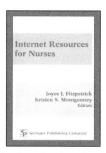

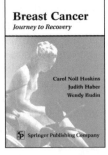

Springer Publishing Company

Modell's Drugs in Current Use and New Drugs, 2001, 47th Edition

Movses Hovsepian, Rph, MS, Editor

Praise for the new edition:

"The forty-seventh edition lives up to the standard that I have come to expect for this extremely useful reference. As a practical tool for the busy clinician, [it] provides a no-nonsense approach to basic drug information when time is of the essence. Compared to other compendiums, the book is more complete, concise, and economical."
—**Barry Goldstein,** RPh, MPA
Directory of Pharmacy Services, NYU Medical Center

Praise for the earlier editions:

" ... keep at hand for fast and easy reference."
—**Journal of the American Pharmaceutical Association**

" ... an excellent reference book."
—**Journal of the American Association of Nurse Anesthetists**

This annually updated drug reference provides succinct information on the new drugs of this year and on medications in current use. It offers a concise and portable alternative to the "mega" drug references available elsewhere—in a compact format that contains essential information on nearly 1,100 generic drugs, with cross references to over 1,200 trade names. Highlights include a glossary listing of common side effects and expanded drug patient care implications for nurses and other allied health professionals.

Contents: Preface
• **Part I:** Old Drugs, New Dosages
• **Part II:** New Drugs
• **Part III:** Glossary of Side Effects

2001   360pp   0-8261-1396-6   softcover

536 Broadway, New York, NY 10012-3955 • Tel: (212) 431-4370 • Fax: (212) 941-7842
Order Toll-Free: (877) 687-7476 • **Order On-Line:** *www.springerpub.com*

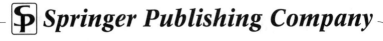

Springer Publishing Company

Nursing Leadership Forum

Editor: **Harriet R. Feldman,** PhD, RN, FAAN
Consulting Editor: **Joyce J. Fitzpatrick,** PhD, RN, FAAN, MBA

Nursing Leadership Forum is a quarterly journal designed for the nurse who leads or aspires to lead in a variety of settings — with patients and families, with nursing staff, in health care or academic institutions, or in the larger community. Within this broad context, the journal explores the ethics, values, and theories underlying the exercise of nursing leadership, as well as innovative ideas for leadership effectiveness.

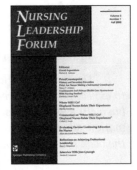

Leadership — once concentrated among the upper echelons of nurses in academia, leading professional organizations, and elite practice settings —has evolved to encompass an entirely new range of challenges. _Nursing Leadership Forum_ captures today's vibrant concept of leadership in its multivariate forms and keeps its readers aware of new ideas and trends.

Each issue of _Nursing Leadership Forum_ features a range of articles, from research presentations to thought-provoking personalized accounts. Book reviews, interviews with colleagues, and a letters column are also a vital part of each issue.

Sample Articles:

- Point: Primary and Secondary Prevention: Are Nurses Making a Substantial Contribution? _Nancy T. Artinian_
- Counterpoint: Isn't Primary Health Care Synonymous With Nursing Practice? _Kimberly Adams-Davis_
- Where Will I Go? Displaced Nurses Relate Their Experiences _Martha Greenberg_
- Evaluating On-Line Continuing Education for Nurses, _Alicia Huckstadt and Karen Hayes_
- Reflections on Achieving Professional Leadership, _Joyce J. Fitzpatrick_
- Interview with Joan Lynaugh, _Sandra B. Lewenson_

Abstracted in: CINAHL, International Nursing Index/MEDLINE, Sociological Abstracts, Social Planning/Policy Development Abstracts

Volume 5 (2000/2001) • 4 Issues • 1076-1632

536 Broadway, New York, NY 10012-3955 • Tel: (212) 431-4370 • Fax: (212) 941-7842
Order Toll-Free: (877) 687-7476 • **Order On-Line:** _www.springerpub.com_